Ethical and Legal Dilemmas
in Occupational
Therapy

SECOND EDITION

RETU

Diana M. Bailey EdD, OTR, FAOTA

Associate Professor
Boston School of Occupational Therapy
Tufts University
Medford, MA

Sharan L. Schwartzberg EdD, OTR, FAOTA

Professor and Chair
Boston School of Occupational Therapy
Tufts University
Medford, MA

F.A. DAVIS | Philadelphia

F. A. Davis Company
1915 Arch Street
Philadelphia, PA 19103
www.fadavis.com

Copyright © 2003 by F. A. Davis Company

Printed in the United States of America

Last digit indicates print number: 10 9 8 7 6 5 4 3 2 1

Acquisitions Editor: Margaret Biblis
Developmental Editor: Thomas J. Robinson
Cover Designer: Louis J. Forgione

Library of Congress Cataloging-in-Publication Data

Ethical and legal dilemmas in occupational therapy / [edited by] Diana M. Bailey, Sharan
  L. Schwartzberg.—2nd ed.
    p. cm.
  Includes bibliographical references and index.
  ISBN 0-8036-1101-3 (alk. paper)
    1. Occupational therapy—Moral and ethical aspects. 2. Occupational therapy—Law and legislation—United States. 3. Occupational therapists—Professional ethics. 4. Occupational therapy—Decision making. I. Bailey, Diana M., 1942- II. Schwartzberg, Sharan L.

RM735.4.E78 2003
174'.2—dc21

2003043575

Preface

We are thrilled that our "little book on ethics" has such a loyal following that we have been asked to write a second edition. The goal of this edition remains the same as the first: to present ethical and legal dilemmas typically faced by occupational therapists, whether they are students, clinicians, or managers. We have added three new topics, following the suggestions of our readers. These topics arise often enough to be worthy of inclusion. The new topics include (1) informed consent when a practitioner is asked for research information concerning his or her clients, (2) confidentiality during group work, and (3) ethical issues to consider when the practitioner is a whistleblower.

The book is still arranged in three sections:

1. The student
2. The clinician
3. The manager

We have maintained the format for the chapters: A vignette describes an ethical dilemma faced by an occupational therapist, and an expert on that issue has responded to the case. The experts have delineated the main areas of concern that practitioners should consider when faced with a similar situation. Penny Kyler has then responded to the experts' comments, bringing to light occupational therapy issues contained in the vignettes and summarizing a process for thinking through a course of action. Penny Kyler is using the same format for case analysis and resolution that she and Ruth Hansen developed several years ago:

- Who are the players in the dilemma?
- What other facts or information are needed?
- What actions might be taken?
- What are the possible consequences of each action? (Hansen, Kamp, & Reitz, 1988)

At the end of each chapter, study questions are included to help the reader integrate the material, and we have added boxes to this edition to highlight important points in the text.

We have invited many of the same contributors to write for this edition and have added a few new people. We are confident that they truly are experts in their field and believe you will find their comments informative and interesting. Once again, we offer their biographies for your information.

Diana M. Bailey, EdD, OTR, FAOTA

Diana Bailey is Associate Professor at Tufts University—Boston School of Occupational Therapy. She is on the Institutional Review Board of the Tufts University School of Arts and Sciences, and in the past has been a member of the institutional review boards of the Gaebler Children's Center and the Walter E. Fernald State School. She has taught about ethical issues for many years. Dr. Bailey has presented at local, state, national, and international workshops and conferences, and has published extensively in occupational therapy.

Norman Daniels, PhD

Norman Daniels is currently Professor of Ethics and Population Health, Department of Population and International Health, Harvard School of Public Health. At the time of participating in writing a chapter in this book, he was Professor in the Philosophy Department at Tufts University. He has written widely on the philosophy of science, ethics, political and social philosophy, and medical ethics. He has lectured and consulted in the United States and abroad on issues of justice and health policy for the United Nations and the President's Commission for the Study of Ethical Problems in Medicine. Recently, he served as a member of the Ethics Working Group that advised President Clinton's Health Care Task Force.

Ezekiel Emanuel, MD, PhD

Ezekiel Emanuel is currently Director of the Clinical Bioethics Center at the National Institute of Health. At the time of participating in writing a chapter in this book, he was a medical ethicist in the Program in Ethics and the Professions at Harvard University and an oncologist at the Dana Farber Cancer Institute. He has written extensively about medical ethics, including a book entitled *The ends of human life: Medical ethics in a liberal polity* (Cambridge, 1991).

Mary Evenson, MS, OTR

Mary Evenson has been the Academic Fieldwork Coordinator at Tufts University—Boston School of Occupational Therapy since 1994. She has extensive experience in administering fieldwork opportunities for students, regularly addressing matters of privacy and confidentiality, in concert with professional standards and legal issues. Ms. Evenson has published on occupational therapy fieldwork and has presented workshops at local, state, national, and international conferences.

Nina Fieldsteel, PhD

Nina Fieldsteel is on the faculty of the Center for Psychoanalytic Studies at the Massachusetts General Hospital, Harvard Medical School Department of Psychiatry. She was previously faculty, senior supervisor, and training analyst at the Postgraduate Center for Mental Health, New York City. Nationally, she has conducted many workshops on ethics and has served on the ethics committee of the American Psychological Association. She is founding editor of *Group: The Journal of the Eastern Group Psychotherapy Society.*

Colin B. Gracey, DMin

Colin Gracey is an Episcopal Chaplain at Northeastern University, where he serves on the Institutional Review Board. He has served as a community representative on the institutional review boards of the Spaulding Rehabilitation Hospital and the Brigham and Women's Hospital. He is a member of the Brigham and Women's panel of the Human Research Committee and the hospital's Continuing Review panel of Partners HealthCare System in Boston, Massachusetts.

Thomas G. Gutheil, MD

Thomas Gutheil, a graduate of Harvard College and Harvard Medical School, is currently Associate Director of Medical Student Training and Co-Director of the Program in Psychiatry and the Law, Massachusetts Mental Health Center. He is also Professor of Psychiatry, Harvard Medical School; former Visiting Lecturer, Harvard School of Law; Special Consultant to the Risk Management Foundation of the Harvard Medical Institutions; and Affiliate Member, Boston Psychoanalytic Society and Institute.

Jim Hinojosa, PhD, OT, FAOTA

Jim Hinojosa is Professor and Chair of the Department of Occupational Therapy in the Steinhardt School of Education at New York University. He served as chair of the Council on Continuing Competence for Occupational Therapy and on the Executive Board of the American Occupational Therapy Association as chair of the Commission on Practice. Dr. Hinojosa has co-authored numerous publications and conducted workshops on issues related to pediatric occupational therapy theory and practice.

Barbara L. Kornblau, JD, OTR

Barbara Kornblau is an attorney and an occupational therapist. She is President of the American Occupational Therapy Association and a professor at Nova Southeastern University in Fort Lauderdale, Florida. She consults with businesses, universities, attorneys, hospitals, state and local governments, and industry about compliance strategies for the Americans with Disabilities Act. She has lectured nationally and internationally and written extensively on legal and ethical issues in rehabilitation.

Penny Kyler, MA, OTR, FAOTA

Penny Kyler is a Public Health Analyst with the Genetic Services Branch, Division of Children with Special Health Needs at the Maternal and Child Health Bureau of the Health Resources and Services Administration. Her responsibilities include consumer education, allied health professional education, and bioethics. Before this position, she was responsible for the ethics office of the American Occupational Therapy Association. Ms. Kyler was honored as one of the *2002 Distinguished Black Marylanders* by Towson University for her work on ethics. She has also recently been elected to the Board of Directors for the American Occupational Therapy Association.

Sally Poole, MA, OT, CHT

Sally Poole is Clinical Assistant Professor in the Steinhardt School of Education at New York University. She is a Certified Hand Therapist and co-owner of Hands-on Rehab in Westchester County, New York, and has worked in the specialty of hand and upper-quadrant rehabilitation since 1979. She has lectured nationally and internationally on hand and upper-quadrant rehabilitation.

Milton Schwartzberg, JD

Milton Schwartzberg has been engaged in the private practice of law in the Boston area since 1974. He has practiced in the fields of litigation, corporate law, and the representation of various business interests. He has represented both individuals and companies in business/employment law controversies. He has also served as legal counsel to automobile dealers and trade associations as well as an arbitrator before the American Arbitration Association. Mr. Schwartzberg's practice has focused on drafting and interpreting contracts in diverse business, corporate, and employment settings.

Sharan L. Schwartzberg, EdD, OTR, FAOTA

Sharan Schwartzberg is Professor and Chair of Tufts University—Boston School of Occupational Therapy. She has written extensively on group work in occupational therapy and presented her ideas both nationally and internationally. Her research also includes interactive reasoning in occupational therapy, and she recently published a book on the topic. Dr. Schwartzberg has taught group process in occupational therapy for 30 years and has conducted research on the efficacy of the Howe and Schwartzberg's Functional Approach to Group Work.

Scott A. Trudeau, MA, OTR

Scott Trudeau is currently a research project director in the Nursing Department of Boston College and a lecturer at Tufts University— Boston School of Occupational Therapy. His work focuses on the care of the elderly, particularly those with progressive dementia. Mr. Trudeau has held a variety of clinical and administrative positions in mental health and long-term care settings and has written and offered workshops in those areas.

Acknowledgements

A sincere thank you goes out to the reviewers:

Roxie M. Blake, MS, OTR/L
Program Director/Assistant
  Professor
Occupational Therapy
University of Southern Maine
Lewiston, ME

Kenneth G. Dechman, MA,
  OTR/L
Rehabilitation Supervisor
Occupational Therapy
Sunnyview Hospital and
  Rehabilitation
Ghent, NY

Karin Opacich, PhD, MPHE,
  OTR/L, FAOTA
Program Director
Occupational Therapy
Opacich Consulting Services
Chicago, IL

Kerstin Potter, MS, OTR/L
Program Director
Occupational Therapy Assistants
Harcum College
Bryn Mawr, PA

Sharon Reitz, PhD, OTR/L,
  FAOTA
Chairperson/Associate Professor
Occupational Therapy
Towson University
Towson, MD

Teepa Snow, MS, OTR/L, FAOTA
Program Director
Occupational Therapy Assistant
Durham Technical Community
  College
Durham, NC

Mary P. Taugher, PhD, OT,
  FAOTA
Assistant Professor
Occupational Therapy
University of Wisconsin
Milwaukee, WI

Donald Walkovich, MS, OTR/L
Chairman/Assistant Professor
Occupational Therapy
St. Francis College
Loretto, PA

Contents

Preface   iii
Acknowledgements   ix

Chapter 1 Theoretical Background   1

Ethical Dilemmas   2
Legal Dilemmas   4
Ethical Principles   4
Legal Principles   9
Conclusion   10
Study Questions   11

Section 1 THE STUDENT   13

Chapter 2 Family Educational Rights and Privacy Act   15

CASE: Parent Demands Rights for Student Found Cheating   15
Expert Commentary   16
Introduction and Update   16
Expert Commentary, Edition 1, 1995   21
Family Educational Rights and Privacy Act   22
University Legal Counsel   23
Other Parties Involved   24
Internal Investigation and Records   26
Department of Education Involvement   27
Conclusion   28
Ethical Commentary   28
Format for Case Analysis and Resolution of Ethical Dilemmas   28
What is a Dilemma?   29
The Case Study Format   29
Student Reported Cheating   30

Summary   33
Study Questions   33

Chapter 3 Section 504 and Americans with Disabilities Act   34

CASE 1: A Student with Emotional Problems
      on Fieldwork Placement   34
CASE 2: A Student with a Physical Disability
   on Fieldwork Placement   35
Expert Commentary   36
Purpose of the Americans with Disabilities Act   36
Section 504 of the Rehabilitation Act   37
The Americans with Disabilities Act   39
Relationship of Ethics to Law   44
Ethical Analysis   45
Case 1: A Student with Emotional Problems
      on Fieldwork Placement   46
Case 2: A Student with a Physical Disability
      on Fieldwork Placement   49
Conclusion   52
Ethical Commentary   53
Cases 1 and 2: Students with a Disability
      on Fieldwork Placements   53
Study Questions   57

Chapter 4 Gates into Practice   58

CASE: Affiliating Fieldwork Student Believes She Is Infected
   with HIV   58
Expert Commentary   59
Evolving Epidemic   59
The Role of the Academic Fieldwork Coordinator   61
Confidentiality   62
Initial Determination: Emotional Stability   63
Testing for HIV   64
Guideline Review   66
Former Client Contact   75
Graduation Ceremony   75
Summary   76
Acknowledgements   77
Ethical Commentary   78
Conclusion   80
Study Questions   80

Section 2 THE CLINICIAN 83

Chapter 5 Functions of the Client Record 85

CASE 1: Documentation for Reimbursement 85
CASE 2: Insurance Dictating Treatment 86
CASE 3: Note Signing 86
Expert Commentary 87
The Roles of the Record 87
Approaches to Documentation 88
Pitfalls of Documentation 89
Signatures and Record-Keeping 91
Conclusion 92
Ethical Commentary 92
Case 1: Documentation for Reimbursement 92
Case 3: Note Signing 95
Study Questions 96

Chapter 6 Modalities and Domain of Practice 97

CASE: Ultrasound Intervention 97
Expert Commentary 98
Introduction 98
Physical Agent Modalities 99
Do Physical Agent Modalities Fall Within The Scope of Practice
  of Occupational Therapy? 100
Do Occupational Therapy Practitioners Have The Educational
  Background to Support The Use of Physical Agent Modalities? 103
When are Occupational Therapy Practitioners Competent to Use
  Physical Agent Modalities? 105
Is It Legal for Occupational Therapy Practitioners to Use Physical
  Agent Modalities? 107
Summary 107
Ethical Commentary 108
Study Questions 111

Chapter 7 Omnibus Budget Reconciliation Act 112

CASE: Restraints in the Nursing Home 112
Expert Commentary 113
Introduction 113
Regulations Governing Nursing Home Care 113
Patterns of Restraint Use 117
Clinical Decision Making 118

Conclusion   119
Ethical Commentary   120
Study Questions   123

Chapter 8 Confidentiality in Groups: Ethical Dilemmas
  and Possible Resolutions   124

CASE: Caregiver Support Group   124
Expert Commentary   125
Introduction   125
Dilemmas Related to the Structure of the Group   126
The Dilemmas Presented by the Incident in the Cafeteria   128
Ethical Dilemmas Created by the Events in the Group   129
Summary   130
Ethical Commentary   130
Conclusion   132
Study Questions   132

Section 3 THE MANAGER   133

Chapter 9 Rationing of Treatment   135

CASE 1: Triage in an Elder Care Facility   135
CASE 2: Too Many Cases to Handle   136
CASE 3: The Seven-Day Work Week   136
Expert Commentary   137
Case 1: Triage in an Elder Care Facility   138
Case 2: Too Many Cases to Handle   145
Case 1: Triage in an Elder Care Facility   148
Case 3: The Seven-Day Work Week   149
Study Questions   151

Chapter 10 Patient Rights: Informed Consent, Competence,
  and the Right to Refuse Treatment   152

CASE 1: Bipolar Disorder and ARC   152
CASE 2: Family Imposes Treatment on Relative   153
Expert Commentary   153
Informed Consent   153
Competence   154
The Emergency Exception   155
The Right to Refuse Treatment   155
Other Rights of Patients   157
Case Scenarios   157
Ethical Commentary   159
Case 1: Bipolar Disorder and ARC   159
Case 2: Family Imposes Treatment on Relative   160
Study Questions   163

Chapter 11 Informed Consent in Research 164

CASE: Therapist Has Questions About Informed Consent 164
Expert Commentary 165
The Common Rule 166
Institutional Resources to Educate, Help, and Guide 166
Regulations Relevant to the Case 167
Stakeholders 167
The Principal Investigator's Request 168
Medical Data Access and Privacy/Confidentiality 168
What Will Guide the Occupational Therapy Practitioner? 169
Dealing With a Perception Gap 171
When "No" is the Way to Go 171
An Educational Moment 172
Slippery Slope and Possible Consequences 172
Reasons for Diligence 173
Ethical Commentary 173
Study Questions 175

Chapter 12 Contracts and Referrals to Private Practice 176

CASE: Absence of a Written Contract 176
Introduction and Update 177
Expert Commentary 177
Expert Commentary, Edition 1, 1995 177
Contracts and Contract Law 178
Conduct Vis-à-vis Elements of a Contract 180
Conclusions 183
Clarity of Contract 184
Ethical Commentary 185
Study Questions 188

Chapter 13 The Whistleblower 189

CASE: The Whistleblower 189
The Role of the Whistleblower 190
Protections 191
Retaliations 192
Support Strategies 192
Ethical Commentary 193
Conclusion 195
Study Questions 195

Glossary 197

References 203

Additional Reading 209

Index 211

Chapter **1**

Theoretical Background

Key Terms

Bioethics
Ethical dilemmas
Ethics

Legal dilemma
Moral development

Consider these scenarios:

A client of yours has had hand surgery but is not making good progress. Her surgeon has a poor reputation in the clinic. One day the client says to you, "I don't feel I am getting better. Was my surgeon any good?" What should you say?

Or:

Your boss tells you that your department must take on a heavier caseload next month because the hospital is opening a burn unit. You will not be given any more staff, and you know that the extra clients will compromise treatment. What should you do?

Or:

An insurance company will not pay a bill because it does not reimburse for the code that has been assigned. Your boss asks you to change the code to one that is reimbursable because the client cannot afford to pay and needs further treatment. What should you do?

These cases illustrate that in occupational therapy, just as in other healthcare professions, many occasions arise in which the practitioner is faced with an ethical or legal dilemma.

We are often poorly prepared to make a decision about what action to take. Sometimes a right or wrong approach is obvious, but more often, when faced with a true dilemma, no clear right path is discernible. We must make a choice between two less-than-perfect actions. This book is about those moments.

We present specific dilemmas faced by occupational practitioners—dilemmas that have actually happened. Then we present experts who offer ethical or legal principles that might guide our actions in that particular situation. We hope that reviewing some actual examples and thinking through possible responses will better prepare practitioners to handle future dilemmas.

Ultimately, we are on our own when it comes to making moral or ethical decisions on the job. One can be told what to do by superiors, but in the long run one must to live with the actions one has taken. All too often, decisions have to be made on the spur of the moment, without time to debate with ourselves or others. Speedy, ill-thought-out decisions lead to anxiety and perhaps later regrets.

Our history, upbringing, and cultural mores will lead us toward an initial decision, one that is predicated on emotional processes. Practitioners who add knowledge to the emotional processes that trigger knee-jerk reactions are better prepared to make reasonable decisions and to reduce the resulting anxiety. In other words, one can enhance how one acts during these difficult moments by thinking about ethical and legal principles ahead of time. Gathering information about challenging issues and viewing those issues from several perspectives will facilitate the decision-making process in the heat of the moment. Practitioners who behave ethically are those who work through their ethical or legal dilemmas by developing a style of decision making. They consider all of the facts, carefully reflect on their options, take advised positions, and are able to tolerate the resulting reactions from others.

There has been much interest in **moral development** since Kohlberg (1963, 1964, 1969) initiated his work in the early 1960s. He analyzed children's and adults' responses to dilemmas and identified stages of moral reasoning. Kohlberg believed: "In the earliest stages, moral reasoning is based on external forces, such as the promise of reward or the threat of punishment. At the most advanced levels, moral reasoning is based on a personal, internal moral code and is unaffected by others' views or society's expectations" (Kail, 1998, p. 310). Gilligan (1982) later presented a different construction of moral understanding—one from the perspective of women. In her analysis of moral development, the relationship is primary. Thereby she differs from Kohlberg, who emphasizes understanding the human rights of the individual. Gilligan's emphasis is on the morality of responsibility through connections between people. Most recently, however, little evidence has been found to support the claim that differences in moral orientation exist between woman and men—that a "care orientation" is predominantly used by women and a "justice orientation" is predominantly used by men (Jaffee & Hyde, 2000).

Ethical Dilemmas

An **ethical dilemma** exists when no single obvious satisfactory choice or answer is appropriate for a certain situation, or when there are only less-

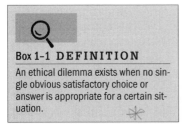

Box 1-1 DEFINITION

An ethical dilemma exists when no single obvious satisfactory choice or answer is appropriate for a certain situation.

than-satisfactory alternatives. On the other hand, we are often faced with difficult situations involving ethical principles in which we can clearly see how we should and should not respond. At these moments, although we might struggle to respond in the "right" manner, in this book these are not considered ethical dilemmas because there is a "right"

response. In the true ethical dilemma, all responses are considered at least partly "wrong" or less than satisfactory by some of the participants.

Ethics

Ethics is a branch of applied philosophy and is a careful and systematic study of the nature of morality. Morality is a set of guidelines and stan-

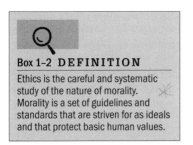

Box 1-2 DEFINITION

Ethics is the careful and systematic study of the nature of morality. Morality is a set of guidelines and standards that are striven for as ideals and that protect basic human values.

dards that are striven for as ideals, to protect basic human values. People's values give direction to the human community and become their moral judgment. Thus people judge (1) conduct or actions as right or wrong, (2) character traits as good or bad, and (3) motives as praiseworthy or blameworthy. The study of ethics goes beyond the law, which deals solely with conduct. Although many occupational therapy ethical dilemmas concern issues

such as finances and education, the focus of most practitioners' dilemmas is their clinical practice. These issues fall under bioethics.

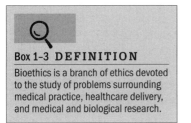

Box 1-3 DEFINITION

Bioethics is a branch of ethics devoted to the study of problems surrounding medical practice, healthcare delivery, and medical and biological research.

Bioethics

Bioethics is a branch of ethics devoted to the study of problems surrounding medical practice, healthcare delivery, and medical and biological research.

Bioethics is a field that has blossomed in recent years from its roots in the early 1960s, partly because of rapid

progress made in the ability to save and prolong life. Quality of life has now become an issue, and bioethicists are called on to examine actions that may lead to a compromised existence. Other medical issues such as surrogate parenthood, HIV and drug testing, and rationing of medical care are some of the issues this generation faces that are unique to the present time and that often lead to ethical dilemmas.

As rehabilitation specialists, occupational therapy practitioners are often caught in these bioethical dilemmas with the rest of the healthcare team. Yet, as individuals, we need to make our own decisions about how we will behave. The growing impact of insurance on patient care, the skyrocketing costs of delivering health care, and the complications of incorporating technical advances in treatment are other factors forcing occupational therapy practitioners to confront ethical dilemmas.

Legal Dilemmas

A **legal dilemma** is one in which a full and equitable solution does not appear to be possible. There is no scientific right or wrong answer. The equities of each argument must be weighed. This is done by discussing one point of view with another point of view, by examining precedents and all sorts of arguments, such as what is good for society and the implications of a ruling. Each Supreme Court judge, for example, has a different view. One judge may look at the letter of the law and another may look to society, depending on the individual judge's orientation.

The law is the collection of rules and regulations by which society is governed. These rules are man-made and regulate social conduct in a formal and binding manner; they reflect society's needs, attitudes, and mores. The established rules and regulations make it easier for people to get along with one another, and these rules affect everyday life, whether or not people realize it.

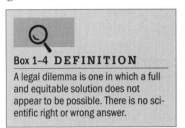

Box 1-4 DEFINITION

A legal dilemma is one in which a full and equitable solution does not appear to be possible. There is no scientific right or wrong answer.

The law is not fixed in place but is a blending of court decisions, state and federal statutes, regulations, and procedures. Interpretations of diverse state laws by different courts or small variations in the circumstances of a case may lead to very different conclusions in two seemingly similar situations. There are no final answers. Law is dynamic—it lives, flows, and changes. No book or set of books, no lawyer or teacher can tell you with complete assurance what is right or wrong or what the final outcome of any case will be.

(Hemelt & Mackert, 1978, p. 3)

Hemelt and Mackert continue graphically: "The law is not the biblical equivalent of the Ten Commandments carved in stone. It is made by society, for society, therefore, it follows logically that the law must change to meet the needs of the particular society for which it is structured" (p. 22).

To form a basis for understanding ethical and legal decision making, some principles that are relevant to healthcare professionals are first presented.

Ethical Principles

Principle of Beneficence

The principle of beneficence comes from the Hippocratic writings and stresses that physicians (in this case, healthcare professionals such as occupational therapy practitioners) have a duty to help. As Munson

Box 1-5 *Summary*

Ethical Principles

Beneficence: Health professionals have a duty to act for the client's good.

Nonmaleficence: "Above all, do no harm."

Utility: Behave in ways that will result in the greatest benefit and the least harm.

Noncomparative justice: People receive that to which they are entitled.

Comparative justice: The application of laws and rules to the distribution of burdens and benefits.

Distributive justice: Is everyone entitled to receive healthcare benefits, and, if so, is everyone entitled to the same amount?

Principle of equality: All benefits and burdens are to be distributed equally.

Principle of need: Goods are parceled out according to individual need; those with greater needs receive a larger portion.

Principle of contribution: Everyone should get back goods in proportion to the amount of his or her productive labor.

Principle of effort: The degree of effort made by the individual should be rewarded by a similar amount of goods.

Principle of autonomy: Rational human beings have the right to be self-determining.

(1988) states: "We should act in ways that promote the welfare of other people" (p. 35). Stated in this context, the occupational therapy practitioner has a duty to act for the client's good. An occasion when this principle is likely to be in peril is when the practitioner takes the role of researcher and the client is a subject in the research. In this situation, the researcher's aim of furthering knowledge may not always be compatible with the practitioner's aim of helping the client.

It is difficult to define the exact limits of beneficence (i.e., what might be a reasonable sacrifice for a practitioner to make for a client) and what is beyond the duty of beneficence. Such a definition is seldom necessary because most of us have fairly clear notions about whether healthcare professionals are fulfilling the duty of beneficence in their actions.

Society is more often made to judge the limits of medical beneficence when deciding on dispensing resources for programs such as Medicare and Medicaid, for prenatal programs, for public clinics, and for medical research and basic science. Such programs are competing for funds with other worthwhile programs, such as defense and housing for the poor, and people often disagree about the boundaries of beneficence. Should all members of society receive all the medical care they need? Are we willing to guarantee a basic level of care only? Should that which is available to the medically insured also be available to the uninsured? Although individual practitioners may feel confident in their ability to judge appropriate parameters for beneficence, they are often caught in the larger web of deciding on the extent of total medical care for our clients.

The American Occupational Therapy Association (AOTA) Code of Ethics (AOTA, 2000a) addresses the issues of beneficence. These issues can be summarized as follows: Occupational therapists must demonstrate concern for the well-being of those receiving their services by

Box 1-6 *By the Law*

The AOTA Occupational Therapy Code of Ethics is a public statement of the values and principles to be used by occupational therapy personnel in promoting and maintaining high standards of behavior in occupational therapy. The Code of Ethics can be found on the AOTA website, www.aota.org, and in the *American Journal of Occupational Therapy* (AOTA, 2000a).

providing services fairly and equitably, by recognizing and appreciating their clients' culture, by establishing fair fees, and by advocating for services needed by their clients.

Principle of Nonmaleficence

The principle of nonmaleficence encompasses the famous moral maxim: "Above all, do no harm." This principle embodies the overriding duty of all healthcare professionals and implies that such things as carelessness, malice, inadvertence, and ignorance should not be allowed to affect the care of clients. Munson's (1988) reformulation of the phrase is: "We ought to act in ways that do not cause needless harm or injury to others" (p. 33). The duty imposed by the principle of nonmaleficence is not a demand to accomplish the impossible because it is generally accepted that there can be no guarantee of correct behavior all the time; however, cautious and diligent behavior can be demanded of healthcare professionals. They can be expected to pay attention and deliberate about each procedure to be used, and they can possess the highest level of knowledge and information relevant to their area of practice. Legally, these are the standards of "due care." By not meeting these standards, healthcare workers open themselves up to moral or legal maleficence.

Certification procedures such as examinations and licensing are used to ensure at least a minimum of knowledge in occupational therapy, but behaviors such as carelessness and haste cannot be legislated against and sometimes lead to inferior client care. Even if no actual harm was caused by such behavior, the practitioner is subjecting the client to unnecessary risk and is violating the standards of due care.

> A failure to act with due care violates the principle of nonmaleficence, even if no harm results, whereas acting with due care does not violate the principle, even if harm does result.
>
> (Munson, 1988, p. 35)

The principle of nonmaleficence is addressed in the AOTA Code of Ethics (AOTA, 2000a). It states that "occupational therapy personnel shall maintain relationships that do not exploit the recipient of services sexually, physically, emotionally, financially, socially, or in any other manner," and ". . . shall avoid relationships or activities that interfere with professional judgment and objectivity" (p. 614).

Principle of Utility

The principle of utility states that "we should act in such a way as to bring about the greatest benefit and the least harm" (Munson, 1988, p.

37). Practitioners need not think of this principle as taking precedence over other principles. For example, practitioners need not take away a client's right to a certain treatment because by doing so they could benefit a group of clients.

The principle of utility is best viewed in conjunction with the principles of beneficence and nonmaleficence. As previously mentioned, the aim of social planning (providing needed yet competing services to the population, such as health care, defense, and bridge building) is to balance the competing needs of society. Taken alone, the principles of beneficence and nonmaleficence are no help in setting priorities. Combined with the principle of utility, these principles enable practitioners to establish an order and a guide for satisfying competing needs. Basically, this principle allows practitioners to use their resources to do as much good as possible. For the clinical manager with limited resources, this principle allows guidelines to be set concerning which clients will be treated, how frequently they will be treated, and with what methods they will be treated (within the constraints of professional standards, facility procedures, and insurance company policies).

Although the principle of utility is not directly addressed in the AOTA Code of Ethics, practitioners are often faced with the dilemma of competing demands. In these instances, practitioners sometimes must decide whom they will and will not treat; whether they will use treatment methods that will allow them to see more individuals, even though those methods might not be best for all the individuals; whether they will offer the optimum number of treatment sessions to those individuals selected for treatment; or whether they will offer fewer treatment sessions to more individuals. Chapter 9 provides a discussion on this thorny issue.

Principles of Distributive Justice

People can and do expect to be treated justly within medicine. If someone arrives at an emergency room with a broken arm before another person with a broken arm, he or she expects to be treated first; however, if someone arrives before a person who is bleeding profusely, he or she expects the bleeding person to be treated first (and would expect the same if the situations were reversed).

There are two major aspects to justice: noncomparative justice, when people receive that to which they are entitled (as in the preceding example), and comparative justice, which is concerned with the application of laws and rules to the distribution of burdens and benefits. The part of comparative justice that is relative to medicine is distributive justice, that which concerns the distribution of medical services. Distributive justice asks: Is everyone entitled to receive healthcare benefits, and, if so, is everyone entitled to the same amount? One way to solve this dilemma is to decide that similar cases ought to be treated in similar ways. First, one must choose what relevant factors are to be considered when deciding whether two cases really are similar. Several theories can help practitioners decide what factors to consider when judging whether cases are similar. Four of these theories can be summarized in the principles of equality, need, contribution, and effort.

According to the principle of equality, all benefits and burdens are to be distributed equally. Everyone is entitled to the same amount, and everyone must bear the load equally. This principle is useful for a society in which there is just enough to go around and not much more, but the principle loses some of its usefulness for an abundant society. The question that arises here is: What about the person who uses greater effort and is most productive? Should this person be rewarded proportionally?

Using the principle of need, goods are parceled out according to individual need; those with greater needs receive a larger portion. This theory is accompanied by the difficulty of deciding what counts as a need. Biologic needs such as food, clothing, and shelter are relatively easy to grasp, but what about emotional or intellectual needs?

Using the principle of contribution, everyone should receive goods in proportion to the amount of his or her productive labor. The difficulty with this principle is that contributions can take forms other than time and labor. For example, some people make intellectual or artistic contributions, whereas others risk money to further a productive venture. How is one type of contribution weighed against another?

According to the principle of effort, the degree of effort made by the individual should be rewarded by a similar amount of goods. Thus the janitor who works hard should be rewarded similarly to the hard-working director, and the lazy person should receive less, regardless of his or her position. This principle appeals to a sense of fairness, but it assumes that everyone has the opportunity to try hard and to do their best. Unfortunately, this is not so because many people are prohibited by circumstances from doing their best work.

Thus all of these theories have problems for execution, and some theorists maintain that a combination of principles of justice must be adopted.

Principle of Autonomy

According to the principle of autonomy, rational human beings have the right to be self-determining. They are acting autonomously when they act on their own choices and decisions. It is often believed that individuals are uniquely qualified to decide what is in their own best interest and that, as such, they have an inherent worth. Others should respect that worth and avoid manipulating them and making decisions for them.

In the healthcare field, there are many opportunities to deny individuals their autonomy (i.e., to restrict the freedom of individuals to act as they might choose). For example, a state law may require that anyone entering a hospital must be screened for the acquired immunodeficiency syndrome (AIDS) virus, or an occupational therapy department protocol may state that all clients who have experienced a cerebral vascular accident must attend a support group. Autonomy is violated in these instances of coercion, even if an individual would have chosen such options if they had been offered.

Another component of autonomy is that of having real options from which to choose. Someone who is poor or uninsured will probably have fewer options in making medical decisions than a wealthy, insured person. Also, people exercise their autonomy in the fullest sense only when they make informed decisions. It is pointless to have options if people are not aware of them, and people are not directing the courses of their own lives if they do not have all the relevant information needed to make a decision. For example, lying to patients about the fact that they have a fatal disease is the ultimate deception because it prevents them from making decisions about how to spend the remainder of their life. Making decisions for "the good" of others without consulting them about their preferences is referred to as paternalism in ethics jargon.

The AOTA Code of Ethics addresses autonomy by stating that practitioners must respect the people they serve by collaborating with them in setting goals and priorities, by informing them of risks and potential outcomes, by respecting their rights to refuse services, by gaining informed consent for research, and by protecting all confidential client communication.

The Code of Ethics contains other principles such as privacy and confidentiality, duty, justice, veracity, and fidelity. Readers may want to obtain a copy of the code because these principles will be referred to later in the text. In addition, the AOTA has published Guidelines to the Occupational Therapy Code of Ethics (1998b) and enforcement procedures for the occupational therapy code of ethics.

Legal Principles

Although legal principles can be consistently applied to healthcare situations, the outcome of the application of these doctrines is often inconsistent.

Box 1-7 *By the Law*

There are Guidelines to the Occupational Therapy Code of Ethics (AOTA, 1998b) designed to indicate a level of expected professional behavior. The guidelines are overarching statements of morally correct action. They can be used for clarification when a perplexing problem arises, as educational or supervisory tools, and to educate the public.

Box 1-8 *By the Law*

The Enforcement Procedures for the Occupational Therapy Code of Ethics (AOTA, 2000b) state: "Any action that is in violation of the spirit and purpose of the Occupational Therapy Code of Ethics is considered unethical. To ensure compliance with the Code, Enforcement Procedures are established and maintained by the [AOTA] Commission on Standards and Ethics" (p. 617).

It should be noted that the AOTA has jurisdiction only over members of the Association in the monitoring and enforcement of the code. The Enforcement Procedures outline disciplinary procedures, investigatory and decision-making procedures; the make-up of the Judicial Council; and an appeal process.

In any medico-legal situation that one will face, one can anticipate having to make judgments. The principle to be followed will be available, but one must select it appropriately to the set of circumstances one encounters.

(Hemelt & Mackert, 1978, p. 22)

The fundamental guiding legal principle in health practice is known as the "reasonably prudent person" theory—namely that a practitioner will do that which a reasonably prudent person would do in the same situation.

The Reasonably Prudent Person Theory

The reasonably prudent person theory is the standard requiring a person to perform a function in a way that any reasonable individual of ordinary prudence, with comparable education, skills, and training under similar circumstances, would perform that same function. This standard has been described as that which requires an individual of ordinary sense to use ordinary care and skill. "Health care practitioners are required to act as similar health care practitioners would in similar circumstances" (Hemelt & Mackert, 1978, p. 29). This concept is simple to grasp, but it is actually extremely difficult to give definite guidelines that would guarantee that a practitioner would not be found negligent or liable if these guidelines were followed. This is because everything is relative to the particular case under review at that particular time.

The healthcare practitioner should remember that one is not judged by the standard expected of the brightest or the least bright health practitioner. He is not judged by what he should have done after reviewing a particular act in hindsight. He is judged on what the average reasonably prudent health practitioner is expected to do faced with a certain set of facts and circumstances and not what one would do two weeks later or after several hours of reflection. The standard is what the reasonably prudent practitioner would be expected to do now, at the particular time, and under the immediate particular circumstances.

(Hemelt & Mackert, 1978, p. 29)

Although no other obvious legal principles have a bearing on the delivery of healthcare services, other items are often considered when there is legal debate regarding health care. These items include custom and usage in the community, accreditation requirements, hospital/facility policy, state licensing standards, and job descriptions. How each of these considerations affects decision making during an ethical dilemma is discussed in the following chapters.

Conclusion

Practitioners will be called on to make moral judgments in their professional lives. When they make sound judgments, they will:

► Have knowledge of the facts
► Try to be impartial
► Try to be clear about the concepts they are using

Practitioners can better anticipate their future responses to ethical and legal dilemmas and prepare themselves to manage these anxious moments by reading, thinking about, and discussing the following cases with their colleagues. If you ask yourself, "What *would* I do in these situations," you will respond from your needs. If you ask yourself, "What *should* I do," you will respond from your values. In the latter instance, you will come closer to making an ethical decision. Working on the Study Questions at the end of each chapter may also assist in developing a model of decision making—a model that considers all of the facts and allows practitioners to adopt well-thought-out positions. If this happens, this book will have achieved its purpose.

Study Questions

1. Identify and describe the following ethics principles:
   a. The principle of beneficence
   b. The principle of nonmaleficence
   c. The principle of utility
   d. The principles of distributive justice
   e. The principle of autonomy

2. How is comparative justice of concern in the distribution of medical services?

3. How is informed decision making different from paternalism?

4. What standard is upheld in the "reasonably prudent person" theory?

5. Describe the elements of an ethical or legal dilemma in occupational therapy and the rationale for studying related principles.

6. Read the following case, and decide which ethical and legal principles apply.

Client Function Versus Discomfort*

Occupational therapist Dr. Nadia Gromsky has been asked by a physician to evaluate a severely deformed infant who is 4 weeks old. The baby has trisomy 13, resulting in a severe cleft lip and palate, multiple deformities of all extremities, and polydactylism. Most children with

---

* Adapted from the New England Occupational Therapy Educators Committee Ethics Workshop: Durham, New Hampshire, 1989.

this condition die within the first year of life, whereas about 20 percent survive beyond 1 year. All are dead by 3 years of age.

Dr. Gromsky recognizes that the child's hand will need to be splinted to ensure structural alignment, to prevent radial deformity, and to allow functional hand use. The parents are reluctant to subject their baby to the discomfort that the splints may cause. Should Dr. Gromsky proceed with the usual recommended therapy?

The Student

S ection 1 begins with a chapter highlighting the Family Educational Rights and Privacy Act. Chapter 3 focuses on Section 504 of the Rehabilitation Act and the Americans with Disabilities Act (ADA). The last chapter in this section, Chapter 4, uses a case scenario of an occupational therapy student who believes she is infected with the human immunodeficiency virus (HIV). Evenson's commentary on Chapter 4 directs the reader's attention to the issues of confidentiality, HIV testing, discrimination, patient protection, professional responsibilities, and the ethical and legal responsibilities of the university and the healthcare setting.

All three chapters focus on the occupational therapy student and the university environment; however, each addresses basic rights of privacy and equality that also apply to practice settings. The student who may be infected with HIV, the student who may have cheated, and students with disabilities all have the right to be treated fairly and equitably. Both attorneys Schwartzberg and Kornblau explain how these rights are protected by federal laws.

Furthermore, the ethical principle of distributive justice applies to each of these situations in the sense that all three students are entitled to educational "goods." In other circumstances, such as in the case of a client, the "goods" may be healthcare resources.

It might be expected that dilemmas would not occur if supervisors, educators, and practitioners acted in accordance with federal and local laws and followed ethical guidelines. Yet, in each of these cases a dilemma does arise. Underlying each situation may be an unconscious bias or perhaps even open prejudice against the student in question. A practical course of action may not be evident because of attitudes or lack of information, resulting in an ethical dilemma to be resolved.

In the treatment of students and clients, ethical principles dictate that occupational therapy practitioners should follow Universal Precautions, protect privacy through confidentiality of records, and provide accommodations for equal access. These directives are particularly evident in the next three chapters.

Chapter 2

Family Educational Rights and Privacy Act

CASE: **Parent Demands Rights for Student Found Cheating**

with commentaries by **Milton Schwartzberg, JD,**
and **Penny Kyler, MA, OTR, FAOTA**

Key Terms

Defamation
Libel
Slander

CASE: Parent Demands Rights for Student Found Cheating

Three graduate students arrive promptly for their appointment with the professor of occupational therapy, who is also the department chair. They stand awkwardly waiting for an invitation to be seated, while expressing apologies for taking time from the busy professor's schedule. After some hesitation, the students report feeling uncomfortable about the visit. They question whether what they have to say is appropriate to raise with the department chair. She encourages them to speak freely without fear of repercussions.

Mary Jo, a student in their class, has been observed evidently cheating by many students on several occasions. They report that she peeks at other student's exam papers and refers to her notes during exams. The students are uncomfortable because they see their visit as "ratting" on a fellow student. Still, they feel that because they are all working very hard and do not cheat, why should Mary Jo get away with this dishonesty? "Someone should know about this and do something about the situation," one student says. The others agree.

The students have not spoken to Mary Jo or to the professor who teaches the course. The department chair acknowledges the seriousness of this situation and encourages the students to confront their peer about the cheating. She also recommends that they come to her office again if Mary Jo's behavior continues. The department chair reports that she will caution students in class about academic dishonesty, that she will again hand out pertinent university policies to all students, and that she will discuss methods of discouraging this behavior with the occupational therapy faculty.

The following day, the department chair receives a phone call from Mary Jo's father. He demands to know exactly what is going on with his daughter. In a loud and aggressive manner, he tells her that he pays his daughter's tuition and that "there are many good lawyers in town who would be interested in this matter, and who will get to the bottom of this. I am not going to let Mary Jo suffer one more minute."

Mary Jo told him that other students have accused her of cheating. She explained that she is dreadfully upset, especially because this comes at a time when her mother is critically ill.

What should the department chair do? Should she discuss this situation further with Mary Jo's father or with the students reporting the incident? She has not yet spoken with Mary Jo or her academic advisor. What are Mary Jo's rights to privacy in the matter? What are the father's or other students' rights? What are the department chair's and the university's rights and obligations in this matter?

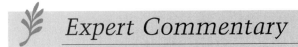

Expert Commentary

By Milton Schwartzberg, JD

Introduction and Update

Since I last wrote about the Family Educational Rights and Privacy Act (FERPA) nearly 10 years ago, there has been a steady evolution of case law and its consequent impact on American academia (Box 2-1). FERPA has developed into the very fabric of American higher education. In so doing, its influence has become pronounced and the involvement of the courts has left an indelible mark on many processes, procedures, and policies that colleges and universities implement when dealing with their students.

Box 2-1 *By the Law*

The Family Educational Rights and Privacy Act (FERPA) is a law designed to protect the privacy of individuals.

Because it would not be possible to review the large number of these cases for this discussion, I have limited my examination to two such cases from opposite sides of the country.

One of the cases has been litigated in the state court system of Washington State. After trial, a jury in Spokane awarded a 1994 graduate of Gonzaga University the sum of $1 million. The plaintiff/former student had sued the university because it had allegedly released private information concerning him to the superintendent of the Washington State public school system. This information concerned the plaintiff's relationship with a special education student. (It should be noted that the student involved indicated that no improprieties took place.) The plaintiff, in addition to alleging violations of FERPA by Gonzaga in releasing the information, also indicated that the school had maintained an erroneous record concerning his performance. Specifically, he indicated that the "concerns" as recorded in his records (and subsequently released to the school superintendent) were wholly unfounded. This claim was supported by the special education student, who never filed any charges with either the authorities or the university. It should be noted that the monetary award given to the plaintiff by the jury was not directly for violations of FERPA, but rather for defamation (Box 2-2), invasion of privacy, negligence, and breach of contract, pursuant to the laws of Washington State.

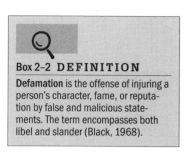

Box 2-2 DEFINITION

Defamation is the offense of injuring a person's character, fame, or reputation by false and malicious statements. The term encompasses both libel and slander (Black, 1968).

Gonzaga University has appealed this finding to the U.S. Supreme Court, which has agreed to hear it. It should be noted that the Supreme Court hears only a small fraction of the cases appealed to it—the vast majority being not considered. Evidently, the Supreme Court considers resolution of this FERPA case and the issues it raises to be of public interest. This appears to be a clear acknowledgment by the highest court in the land that FERPA is not only significant, but its interpretation and implementation in the twenty-first century are also fundamental elements of the relationship between students and higher education.

The University's position in opposing the earlier finding was succinctly stated by its attorney, who told the Supreme Court that if the ruling stands, it "would be contrary to precedent, destructive to the private organization's freedom, and [create] an open floodgate for lawsuits" (*John G. Roberts, Jr. Gonzaga University* v. *Doe*, U.S. Supreme Court Docket No. 01-679). Whether the Court considers Mr. Roberts' argument to be hyperbolic or totally valid remains to be seen. A ruling and written opinion had not been issued at the time this discussion was written. Either way, the issues raised by FERPA and brought up in this case have a great impact on the persons and educational institutions within its jurisdiction, purview, and influence, as *Gonzaga* v. *Doe* has demonstrated.

Another case that has raised serious and volatile issues is one filed in the Massachusetts court system against a renowned institution of higher education. *Shin* v. *Massachusetts Institute of Technology* (M.I.T.) is a wrongful death suit filed by the parents of a 19-year-old M.I.T. sophomore whose suicide came as a complete shock and surprise to her family. Her parents claim that although M.I.T. knew of their daughter's serious and ongoing emotional difficulties, it purposefully withheld all such information from the family.

It is interesting to observe how two different universities located at opposite ends of the country have dealt with the issue of student privacy rights in entirely opposite ways. Gonzaga chose, without prior authorization, to release information to a public agency that it knew or should have known would have an adverse effect on the subject student/graduate seeking employment as a teacher. M.I.T. has just been formally accused of failing to release critical information to the parents of a student who committed suicide. The parents now allege that M.I.T. should have notified them about the multiple instances of self-mutilation and consequent psychiatric treatments that occurred while their daughter was enrolled as a student. They further allege that "M.I.T.'s failure to design and implement an adequate mental health protocol including the effective use of the Family Educational Rights and Privacy Act and parental involvement constitutes a willful, wanton or reckless violation of law resulting in death by suicide of Elizabeth Shin" (*Shin, et al.* v. *M.I.T., et al.*, Middlesex Superior Court (Massachusetts), Civil Action No. 02-0403).

Although the suit does not spell out specifically what constitutes "an effective use of the Family Educational Rights and Privacy Act" in the context of the scenario spelled out by the plaintiffs, several inferences can be made. First, it is clear that the family maintains that M.I.T. and its medical/psychiatric service providers were obligated to inform them of their daughter's self-destructive behavior. Furthermore, the family has indicated that M.I.T.'s failure to include "family involvement" in these circumstances is a contributing factor to their daughter's death. We can infer that the family's position is that had M.I.T. notified them of the multiple instances of their daughter's self-mutilation and psychiatric hospitalizations, she would still be alive today. Taking this line of reasoning one step further, excluding them from this process evidently not only offended the family, but has also now convinced them that this was a factor contributing to their daughter's demise. It should be noted the media has reported that the M.I.T. student, Elizabeth Shin, exhibited serious self-destructive behavior as a high school student while resident with her family. This situation may be brought up by M.I.T. in its defense, claiming the family knew that a serious problem existed with their daughter even before she attended M.I.T.; however, the central issue does remain. To what extent is the university obligated to provide information to the parents of any of its students?

Gonzaga University, on its own initiative, provided information to a governmental agency. Would a suit have been filed if this disclosure had been made to the student's family instead? Probably not because the thrust of this suit dealt with the career damage sustained by the student/graduate as a result of Gonzaga's disclosure. These two cases represent the extremes in how FERPA has been interpreted by American institutions of higher learning in very recent history. Further, whereas the Gonzaga case has been litigated to its finality before the U.S. Supreme Court, the M.I.T. case is in its infancy. Gonzaga has shown that a university has gone much too far when it releases information (on its own initiative) to a governmental agency. This is exacerbated further when the released report disparages the former student and may not, in fact, be accurate. As stated, this student recovered additional damages for defamation and other causes of action as well. The large monetary award underscores the court's finding that Gonzaga's conduct was offensive. Moreover, it was also likely calculated to serve as a deterrent.

American jurisprudence is not in the business of writing laws and statutes. Rather, its mission is to interpret laws and their applicability to given facts and circumstances. In so doing, it is sometimes said that courts "make law." This is not in the literal sense, of course. Rather, by interpreting, striking down, and modifying the laws that Congress, state legislatures, and local municipalities create, courts, in fact, make critical findings. These actions decide whether laws are valid, enforceable, or must be struck down, in whole or in part. This process is actually happening now with respect to FERPA.

When I first examined FERPA for the first edition of this book, it was a relatively new statute. Having been on the books for a limited period, little in the way of judicial review had taken place. In the intervening years, however, FERPA and privacy issues have remained at the forefront of society's concerns. In fact, attempts have been made to expand FERPA-type laws into the areas of medical/health insurance coverage as well as in the areas of personal credit and financial information.

The Gonzaga case has illustrated when an institution of higher learning has gone too far in revealing information. The M.I.T. case, although only recently filed, raises several questions that a judge and jury will ultimately decide. The American system of justice holds that when a jury sits, it alone decides issues of fact. A judge interprets and rules on issues of law. For example, M.I.T. in its defense has claimed that "the Family Educational Rights and Privacy Act provides no private right of action and no basis for liability on the part of any of the defendants." (See: Defendant's Second Affirmative Defense, *Shin, et al.* v. *M.I.T., et al.*, Middlesex Superior Court (Mass.) Civil Action No. 02-0403). Essentially this means that M.I.T. alleges that FERPA does not allow individuals (as opposed to governmental agencies) to prosecute a lawsuit claiming FERPA damages. A judge will decide this issue before the case is tried in front of a jury. Also, although M.I.T. did not raise it in their defense, federal statutes are typically adjudicated in federal as opposed to state courts. These primarily technical issues will be sorted out during the course of litigation long before the jury trial.

It will likely take two to three years before this case is fully tried, and a final determination will take even longer if appeals are made; however, it is not unusual for the parties in a wrongful death suit to settle the case well before trial. In any event, this litigation raises profound issues in the area of the administration of contemporary higher education.

I would now like to return to the scenario in the text of Chapter 2 concerning "Parent Demands Rights for Student Found Cheating." In this analysis, the rights, duties, and obligations of the respective parties were discussed in light of FERPA. Since that time, litigation, both completed and ongoing, is influencing the meaning and application of FERPA. The interpretation has been that one university has gone too far in releasing information, whereas another is accused of not going far enough and thereby contributing to a student's death.

Viewing FERPA in the context of higher education, the original Chapter 2 scenario, and what has transpired since, one is struck by how the roles of the "players" have changed and continue to evolve. Specifically, in taking pains to respect student privacy rights, the university, in so doing, is acknowledging that it is conferring the rights and responsibilities of an adult on the member of its student body. Implicit in this concept is the perception that the student, in turn, will act more responsibly and no longer require the closer supervision and scrutiny that an adolescent would. In returning to the original FERPA scenario, Mary Jo, who was suspected of cheating, could expect to be treated more like an adult and less like an adolescent. This is consistent with a loosening over time of the long-held doctrine of in loco parentis, which is defined as "In the place of a parent; instead of a parent; charged factitiously, with a parent's rights, duties and responsibilities" (Black, 1968).

Before the enactment of FERPA, this doctrine was the clear framework for how a university would define its obligations and duties vis-à-vis its students. In so doing, for all intents and purposes the university was entrusted by a student's family to act as a virtual parental surrogate. Accordingly, the university was free to share information about the student and to confer with the parents. FERPA, as discussed, originally severely restricted this free flow of communication and caused a major structural diminution in the application of the in loco parentis doctrine. Clearly, before FERPA, members of the faculty would be free to confront Mary Jo, discuss the allegations with her parents, and attempt to reach a mutually agreeable course of action. Acting as a surrogate parent, the university would likely impose greater latitude and flexibility to situations involving student indiscretion. Mindful of privacy considerations in the context of a more litigious society, however, the university is likely to consult its attorneys regularly, as suggested in the original first edition text. This is consistent with treating students as "adults" within the context of privacy issues in general and FERPA in particular.

Clearly, the Gonzaga case has shown that disclosures of student information furnished as a result of the university's own initiative violate privacy laws. In fact, as Gonzaga illustrated, the university can also be held liable for other civil wrongs (e.g., defamation) and be forced to pay significant monetary damages. On the opposite spectrum, the Shin family has sued M.I.T. for not providing information, which they claim could have prevented their daughter's suicide. M.I.T. claims that they were honoring their student's specific directive not to contact her parents. Evidently, the family is devastated by the apparent abandonment of all in loco parentis principles by M.I.T. vis-à-vis their daughter. M.I.T., in contrast to Gonzaga, chose not to release or share information concerning this student's mental health difficulties and self-destructive behavior. Is this the direction in which higher education is now moving? Are the privacy rights of students paramount in all situations? The outcome of this ethical (Should the university inform the family in a potentially life-threatening situation?) and legal dilemma (By so doing, it is contrary to a specific directive given by the student and may also violate FERPA.) will likely have far-reaching implications for American higher education. The interpretation and implementation of FERPA are dynamic issues that are constantly evolving. This chapter has briefly discussed its current state, which admittedly will soon change again.

Expert Commentary
Edition 1, 1995

By Milton Schwartzberg, JD

In the early 1970s, this country was winding down the war in Southeast Asia while engaging in a period of profound introspection. This self-examination culminated in the Watergate hearings of 1973 and 1974, which brought down the presidency of Richard Nixon.

These hearings brought the light of public scrutiny on many practices and actions that were distasteful, unethical, and sometimes illegal. What many people found most disturbing was that a multitude of these acts were committed by persons employed by the government and using governmental resources. The motives for these acts were varied; however, the general public reaction was not: Shock, indignation, and even horror were commonplace.

Governmental intrusions into the private lives of Americans achieved increasing notoriety when Congress decided to act. Senator Sam Ervin, of the Watergate Committee, commented on the need for this proposed legislation:

> It seems that now, as never before, the appetite of government and
> private organizations for information about individuals threatens to

usurp the right to privacy which I have long felt to be amongst the most basic of our civil liberties as a free people.

[120 Cong. Rec. 12, 646 (1974)]

Technological advances undoubtedly exacerbated this concern. The ubiquitous computer has become the all-encompassing repository of information about everyone. Abuses in the public sector carried out by government agencies such as the Internal Revenue Service (IRS) and the Federal Bureau of Investigation (FBI) were no doubt on Sen. Ervin's mind when he eloquently gave his unqualified support to this legislation.

FERPA initially was limited to curbing abuses emanating from governmental sources. It soon became clear that invasions of privacy and other noxious intrusions into the lives of Americans were not all instigated by the government. Further legislation provided for coverage into other areas.

Family Educational Rights and Privacy Act

In 1974, FERPA became law. The original Privacy Act, 5 U.S.C. section 552a, sought to restrict the ability of federal agencies to gather, use, and disclose information about individuals. The enactment of FERPA expanded protection of privacy to include educational records and the rights of students to inspect and review these records. Furthermore, FERPA provides for a hearing mechanism designed to correct inaccurate or misleading information contained in these educational records.

FERPA mandates that a college student's records are presumed to be confidential, with certain exceptions. These records may be released to the parents of an undergraduate student if that student is claimed as a dependent for income tax purposes. Some colleges on the undergraduate level presume that this is the case and, in practice, so inform students and their parents; however, such a student may file a statement to the contrary and preserve the confidentiality of his or her records, even from parents.

FERPA provides an exception to confidentiality in what is referred to as "directory information" (Box 2-3). Typically, this includes addresses, telephone numbers, birth dates, fields of study, and other related data. Some institutions have even given students the option of withholding information of this type as well, although it is not clear to what extent this allowance is consistent with FERPA.

Box 2-3 *Summary*

Student Directory Information is a listing that typically includes addresses, telephone numbers, birth dates, fields of study, and other related data.

At the time that FERPA was introduced, Congress felt that the American public strongly desired this type of legislation. With this public mandate in mind, Congress sought to impose the objectives of FERPA onto American higher education. Although some states had previously enacted privacy protection laws, no consistent and broad-ranging legislation dealt specifically with the protection of privacy rights in the academic setting. The existing patchwork-quilt design of state privacy laws added further motivation for Congress to enact FERPA and provide consistency in setting privacy protection standards in American higher education.

FERPA has made a strong impact on academics, particularly academic administrators. By making the availability of federal funding conditional on adherence to this law, the government has effectively put teeth into this legislation. Because higher education—both public and private—largely depends on governmental funding, FERPA is a force to be reckoned with in American academia.

This discussion does not advocate nor state an opinion regarding the imposition of federal standards and regulations in certain aspects of higher education. Rather, it seeks to observe and discuss the impact and influence of this legislation in a real-life higher education vignette.

In the 20 years that FERPA has been in existence, it has been woven into the fabric of American higher education. FERPA has received mixed reviews by academia. Some object to governmental interference at this level as a matter of principle and view it as an unwarranted intrusion. Others see it as a necessity not only in combating invasions of privacy in higher education, but also in establishing structure in place of ambiguous and sometimes conflicting laws and regulations. FERPA gives clearer guidance to academic administrators who are confronted with situations like that described in the previous scenario.

University Legal Counsel

In being presented with the dilemma previously discussed, I would first advise the department chair to contact the university legal counsel. The major reason for this response is that Mary Jo's father has said that he may consider taking legal action. It is in both the department chair's and the university's best interests to deal with Mary Jo's father on an equal footing.

Keep in mind that in this case example, anything the department chair says or does is on behalf of the university. She is legally the university's agent, which means that she is acting on the institution's behalf. Therefore, it is even more imperative to contact university legal counsel. In addition, the institution's legal counsel is in a position to ensure that any response made on its behalf is consistent not only with FERPA but also with university rules, regulations, and policies. Since virtually all institutions of higher learning have specific policies dealing with allegations of unethical conduct of students, these policies must be given serious consideration as well.

At this point, the department chair should act only on advice of counsel. She might also be advised to report this matter to her immediate supervisor, typically an academic dean. A response formulated by legal counsel, with input by the department chair and the dean, would be my advice at this stage. This response is likely to inform Mary Jo's father that discussions of this matter are subject to the provisions of FERPA. Because the father has at least implied taking legal action, he has consequently created an adversarial relationship with the department chair and the university at large. Therefore, I would advise the department chair to deal with Mary Jo's father firmly the next time he calls. She should not discuss details of the alleged cheating, not only because of FERPA considerations, but also so that the university will avoid further potential liability.

If the department chair is uncomfortable dealing directly with Mary Jo's father, her subordinate can direct this call to the university legal counsel. Again, the implied threat of legal suit justifies this course of action.

Other Parties Involved

Mary Jo

The obligations of the department chair must be recalled. First, she is an agent and representative of the university. Second, her actions must take into account the rights of all parties involved. These include Mary Jo, her parents, the other graduate students, and the university. It is difficult to balance these competing and, in this instance, conflicting interests. The department chair or any other university representative should not further discuss the substance of these allegations with Mary Jo's father. Without specific written permission, given by Mary Jo, FERPA would likely prohibit such a communication at this point. As will be discussed, internal investigations within the established university structure do not violate FERPA; however, a discussion with an outside party (even the parent of a graduate student) appears to violate the privacy standards established. It may be suggested to Mary Jo that if she wants her father to intervene or communicate on her behalf in these circumstances, that she first provide the required written permission. If Mary Jo seeks to establish contact with the department chair, however, a potential dilemma may arise.

If Mary Jo threatens or implies legal action such as her father has done, then I think the department chair should refer her to university legal counsel as well. If no threats are made—either express or implied—then the department chair is obligated to treat Mary Jo as she does all students. Note that the options afforded the department chair depend primarily on university policy. Any provisions of university policy dealing with the unethical behavior of students, as well as the existence of a plagiarism or cheating policy at the university, is unknown at this time.

For the purposes of discussion here, assume that the university has a policy prohibiting specific acts of unethical conduct by its students. Such acts would include those of which Mary Jo is accused. These acts are subject to unspecified punishment.

Other Students and Faculty

The department chair at the university must now consider how to deal with the other students. Her authority, as agent of the university, obligates her to conduct herself within the rules and regulations thereof. If she is unclear about the university rules and procedures concerning cheating, she should consult legal counsel. I would advise her to obtain a copy of the university regulations in this area and consider distributing them to all students. She should not conduct any further discussions with other students concerning Mary Jo's alleged cheating. The only exception to this prohibition is if she becomes involved in a formal university investigation or disciplinary proceeding. The department chair should also be careful to whom and under what circumstances she divulges what would be considered "educational records" pertaining to Mary Jo. FERPA, 20 U.S.C. section 32g (b), specifically prohibits dissemination of student education records by educational institutions without written permission.

In addition to "directory information," the limited list of exceptions that permit release without written permission includes releases "to other school officials including teachers within the educational institution or local educational agency who have been determined by such agency or institution to have legitimate educational interests" [20 U.S.C. section 1232g (a)(5)(A)]. Presumably, the internal investigation of the charges against Mary Jo qualifies as being in the latter category of exceptions. At the graduate level of higher education, FERPA requires written permission directly from the student. Parental consent is not acceptable [20 U.S.C. (g)]. This contrasts with the previously mentioned standard at the undergraduate level, wherein dependency claimed by parents for income tax purposes gives them the right to access their child's educational records.

An argument can be made that because the allegations of cheating are unproven, they are not yet part of Mary Jo's educational record. If these allegations are later proven, however, they could eventually become part of Mary Jo's records. FERPA, 20 U.S.C. section 1232g (1)(A), would permit Mary Jo to access these educational records to ensure accuracy.

I would now advise the department chair to disseminate the materials containing university policy regarding cheating. I would also encourage her to discuss the subject of cheating generally with her students and the faculty, with the goal of discouraging this activity. The department chair is obligated to maintain the integrity of the educational process. Having discussions on this subject is certainly appropriate. I would caution the chair not to mention anyone by name and not to encourage this practice in open discussions among the students. As the agent of the university, the department chair speaks for the institution, and she must therefore proceed with caution. The path is lined with potential FERPA, libel, slander, and defamation mines (Boxes 2-4, 2-5). Again, at this stage it would be good practice to involve university legal

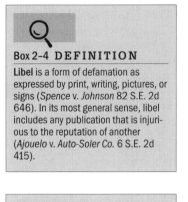

Box 2-4 DEFINITION

Libel is a form of defamation as expressed by print, writing, pictures, or signs (*Spence* v. *Johnson* 82 S.E. 2d 646). In its most general sense, libel includes any publication that is injurious to the reputation of another (*Ajouelo* v. *Auto-Soler Co.* 6 S.E. 2d 415).

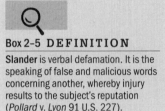

Box 2-5 DEFINITION

Slander is verbal defamation. It is the speaking of false and malicious words concerning another, whereby injury results to the subject's reputation (*Pollard* v. *Lyon* 91 U.S. 227).

counsel. Counsel is in a position to evaluate the merits of each situation and may, in some instances, advise against dissemination of these materials at this time.

Take note of the fact that the university undoubtedly has a written set of policies that form, in effect, a contract between it and the attending students. This policy would determine whether the allegations made against Mary Jo will be investigated and possibly prosecuted.

Because most, if not all, universities have clearly defined policies that do not tolerate cheating or plagiarism of any type, the failure to enforce such a policy against Mary Jo would amount to a breach of contract by the university vis-à-vis the other students. These other students are clearly justified in refusing to tolerate this behavior not only because it is unethical, but also because it cheapens and devalues the entire educational process. It would now be appropriate to assure these students that the matter is being investigated internally pursuant to university policy. They should not confront Mary Jo nor further publicize the matter because they may have to testify at a later hearing.

Internal Investigation and Records

Internal investigations have a legitimate educational purpose. Certainly, the objective of maintaining the integrity of the educational process entitles all those within the university community to discuss the matter of cheating with that goal in mind. In fact, the failure of the university to act now would be harmful in such future instances. By remaining passive in this situation, the department chair and the university become open to future charges of dissemination by selective enforcement. Because integrity is among their most valued components, both the department and the university have no choice but to act.

Remember that it is imperative to allow Mary Jo an appropriate forum to address the charges against her and to defend herself. Although this is not a situation in which Mary Jo's constitutional rights are at stake (because there is no exposure to potential criminal liability), she should be treated fairly and equitably. Any failure to so treat her would make her case stronger if she seeks to later sue the university for defamation, intentional infliction of emotional distress, or other potential causes of action.

In any event, Mary Jo is entitled to challenge the university records maintained in her name by way of a hearing "in order to insure that the records are not inaccurate, misleading or otherwise in violation of the privacy or other rights of students and to provide an opportunity for the correction or deletion of any such inaccurate, misleading or otherwise inappropriate data contained therein and to insert into such records a written explanation" [20 U.S.C. section 1232g (a)(2)]. I would advise the department chair that it is imperative to make Mary Jo aware of her rights under FERPA. Perhaps the university legal counsel could assist in providing this information for Mary Jo. She should be informed that the results of the investigation are not public record and that FERPA prevents their release without her permission.

What is not yet clear under FERPA is whether certain parts of a student's records can be withheld while other parts are disseminated. For example, assume that the outcome of Mary Jo's hearings determined that she did cheat repeatedly, and she was subsequently suspended or expelled from the university. If she wished to attend graduate school elsewhere, could she have her prior records forwarded for consideration yet specifically prohibit the revelation of the detrimental information? Although there is no current case or ruling on this point, I do not believe that it could be done. The practical considerations involved in allowing a student to pick and choose what grades could be released and what would stay sealed, I believe, are not consistent with the aims of FERPA.

Clearly, maintaining privacy rights in the educational setting is sacrosanct under FERPA. If Mary Jo releases her records as described, she does not appear to have the right to censor portions of that record; however, FERPA has charged the Secretary of Education with investigating any FERPA violations via a review board within the Department of Education.

The way the law is currently structured, Mary Jo's rights to privacy and fairness must be rigidly observed. Even though strong evidence suggests that her conduct was repugnant, Mary Jo is in the position of potentially causing the university (and in turn, the department) great harm.

If she contests the finding of an investigation that is adverse to her, the university is faced with potentially costly litigation. According to FERPA, if she contests the way such an adverse ruling is described in her records, another hearing within the university must take place.

Department of Education Involvement

In the event that this hearing renders a ruling that is unsatisfactory to Mary Jo, she can then go further still. She has the option of bringing this matter directly before the Department of Education. She may allege that her FERPA rights to privacy are being violated because her educational records contain what she considers to be erroneous and defamatory information. I believe that eventually these claims would not prevail; however, the intervening period would cause the department chair and the university considerable discomfort because an adverse ruling could potentially cut off federal funding.

Clearly, although FERPA's objectives are noble, there is considerable negative potential that a cynical student could exploit. If such a person regularly resorts to cheating to gain academic advancement, are there any bounds to her self-promotion? Could FERPA be misused by such an individual?

Conclusion

To minimize the possible negative impact of FERPA, it is critical to be aware of its provisions and to scrupulously ensure that they are not violated. I believe it is good practice, particularly in the higher education setting, to consult with university legal counsel on any law impacting academia. I would advise any department chair to ask the university counsel to come to a department meeting to explain FERPA and how to incorporate it into the educational process. Knowledge of FERPA is essential to all those affiliated with the university, even the students.

Finally, I suggest that the department chair and university legal counsel devise a do's and don'ts list regarding FERPA. Although it is impossible to anticipate every conceivable situation that has FERPA implications, one can plan on the more common and frequent instances in which FERPA regulations are of concern in the higher education setting.

There is no reason why the academic community and FERPA cannot peacefully coexist. The privacy rights of students can be respected without jeopardizing federal funding of higher education. A willingness to understand the provisions of FERPA will benefit all those who are affected by this law.

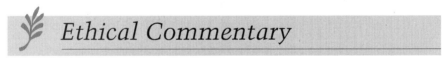

Ethical Commentary

By Penny Kyler, MA, OTR, FAOTA

Commentary on each of the chapters that follow will provide the foundation for certain approaches that may be taken during ethical decision making. Readers will be asked to take a stand for or against an approach and to develop arguments for their decisions.

**Format for Case Analysis
and Resolution of Ethical Dilemmas**

Like most healthcare professionals, occupational therapy practitioners are guided by a professional code of ethics (American Occupational

Therapy Association [AOTA], 2000a) and standards of practice (AOTA, 1998a). The companion documents, Guidelines to the Occupational Therapy Code of Ethics (1998b) and the Core Values and Attitudes of Occupational Therapy Practice statements (AOTA, 1993a), act as reference guides to the code of ethics and provide additional guidance for ethical decision making; however, none of these documents provide methods for resolving dilemmas. Hansen and Kyler-Hutchison (1989) provide a format for case analysis and resolution of ethical dilemmas. Other formats are available, and individuals are encouraged to add or to delete from this particular format. Educators may wish to ask students some additional questions to elicit their understanding of ethics and problem solving. As an example, they may wish to ask students how they incorporate their values and beliefs while they are analyzing problems. When using the Hansen and Kyler-Hutchison format, readers are asked:

1. Who are the players in the dilemma?
2. What other information or facts are needed?
3. What possible actions can be taken?
4. What are the likely consequences (ethical, legal, or medical) of each action?
5. Choose an action you can defend.

What is a Dilemma?

Situations are only defined as dilemmas when two or more right or two or more unsatisfactory solutions exist, not when there is a right judged against a wrong. In the latter situation, the course of action to be taken is generally clear, but the former situations pose a dilemma.

More specifically, moral dilemmas are created by conflicting moral principles. Several actions may be seen as morally correct, even though it may be possible to justify one action to a greater degree than the others. By the same token, it is possible for two individuals to take opposing courses of action and that both of those actions are justifiable. Ideally, the moral action an individual takes is based on the application of ethical principles. Those principles guide the individual and provide the rationale for action. Ethics theory informs us that these principles include beneficence, utility, distributive justice, duty, veracity, autonomy, and others, as discussed in Chapter 1.

The Case Study Format

The cases at the beginning of each chapter will help readers reflect on their values in regard to client care. It is hoped that using the format in the commentary sections to analyze the cases will help readers develop skill in moral reasoning and decision making.

Student Reported Cheating

In this chapter on FERPA, Attorney Schwartzberg has written on the legal procedures and the current legal precedents available for FERPA. One should consider the ethical issues as well as the legal issues while resolving the dilemmas raised by a student who is cheating. Besides the legal concerns articulated by Attorney Schwartzberg, several ethical issues must also be considered, such as trust and honesty.

Occupational therapy practitioners subscribe to several core values. These values are a combination of moral development and professional commitment. The basic value that is in jeopardy in the case of Mary Jo is the value of trust. For practitioners to develop a therapeutic alliance with clients or to enter a pedagogic relationship with students, a sense of trust has to exist. Trust is the basis of student (or client) reliance on the integrity, ability, and character of the professor (or practitions). People who are trusted generally inspire confidence and are expected to be truthful, regardless of the situation. When students do not feel trust, their confidence in professors is shaken. Confidence is necessary to permit students to progress in their education. Principle 6 of the Occupational Therapy Code of Ethics, *veracity*, notes that practitioners should refrain from using or participating in any form of false, fraudulent, deceptive, or unfair statements. These concepts must be considered when dealing with the students who are reporting the cheating and the student accused of cheating. What are the facts?

Who Are the Players?

It is easy to determine that the three graduate students, Mary Jo, all of the occupational therapy students, all of the students' families, the faculty, and the department chair are the players. Because this situation takes place in an academic environment, however, other individuals or offices may be involved, including the dean, the student relations office, and the university legal counsel. Because Mary Jo is going out into practice, the players may also include potential employers, clients, payers, and other students not in this occupational therapy program. Which other players would you include?

What Other Information Is Needed?

What are the histories of all involved—social and educational? What has been the ongoing relationship between Mary Jo and her classmates? What are the university's policies and procedures on cheating? Does the occupational therapy department or the university have an honor code? Is there a process other than going to the department chair that addresses this issue? Has the AOTA Code of Ethics been taught in the curriculum? Is it mentioned in admissions information? What is the relationship between the faculty and students? What type of relationship does Mary Jo have with her parents? What other behaviors of Mary Jo, if any, have been noticed by the faculty and students? Are the three reporting students being honest? What is their motivation? What other information would you seek?

What Actions May Be Taken and What Are the Possible Consequences?

Following are some ideas to initiate a thought process and to spark debate about this case:

1. What are the possible outcomes of this case of alleged cheating? A ripple effect could occur that would limit faculty interaction with students. Mary Jo may be ostracized by her peers, which could have an effect on learning in the general milieu. The collaborative process between faculty and students could break down, which would alter teaching methods and student assignments.
2. Most faculty–student and practitioner–client relationships are based on a foundation of trust and collaboration. Mary Jo's act of cheating raises the questions of how much she can be trusted and what other potentially self-serving acts she might exhibit in the future, once she is an occupational therapy practitioner.
3. A perspective for the faculty to consider regarding this case is that of pausing to reflect on the code of ethics and core values of occupational therapy. Have these values been discussed with the students? Are they integrated into occupational therapy courses throughout the curriculum? Have the faculty members determined how to garner a greater understanding and appreciation of the code of ethics and core values of occupational therapy? Have the faculty members studied the principles and evaluated which values the students are and are not consistently demonstrating? If there is not a school of occupational therapy ethics code or pledge, could developing one be part of a class assignment?
4. Regarding FERPA, many faculty and staff members have not been educated about what FERPA does and does not require. A training session with the university legal counsel regarding the provisions of FERPA could be part of a faculty meeting.
5. Students and faculty members may wish to look at the triad of legal, professional, and academic parameters. What are the functions of professional ethics? How do the professions of law, education, and occupational therapy compare and contrast regarding honor codes? What impact does a breech of a school honor code have on the potential to practice one's profession? If students are preparing to join a profession, should they be held accountable to a higher standard than those expected of other students?

Box 2-6 ON THE WEB

The Website for the NBCOT is www.nbcot.com. The *NBCOT Summer and Fall 2002 Candidate Handbook* may be viewed at www.proexam.org/nbcot/047-hand.pdf.
The Handbook states the following practitioner responsibilities under Examination Content Areas (pp. 25, 27):

G. **Responsibilities as a professional**
   Knowledge and skills related to:
1. occupational therapy roles, code of ethics, and standards of practice
2. federal, state, and local regulations governing occupational therapy practice

6. The issue of "the greater good" is also important to consider. The negative impact of Mary Jo's action on a group of individuals is considerable. Also, the indication that this episode of cheating was not an isolated incident for Mary Jo should be considered in the larger context of her total school and professional career. It should be noted that the National Board for Certification in Occupational Therapy (NBCOT), as well as many licensure boards, require verification of a student's good character (Box 2-6). NBCOT mentions the topic both in the Candidates Handbook and when a student sits for the examination and signs an attestation that the student applicant will abide by the AOTA Occupational Therapy Code of Ethics (Personal communication, T. LaGarde, June 2002).

7. In debating the case of Mary Jo, consider whether the students in the case have a chance to bring their values to bear in determining what actions should be taken. The informative model of ethical decision making (Emanuel & Emanuel, 1992) suggests that the faculty member should provide the students with all of the relevant facts and options so that they can decide which action should be taken. The faculty member helps with the implementation of the decision. This model is weighted heavily toward autonomous decision making; and although it takes a moral high ground, it also allows for the possibility that an individual might make a decision that others would not like. The informative model is in keeping with the spirit of FERPA in that it endorses informed decision making. The faculty member is seen as a technical expert, and the student has choice and control over the outcome. Shared decision making constructed around information, participation, and respect would allow all players in Mary Jo's case to evaluate available courses of action, express concerns and wishes, and make an ideal decision.

Summary

With the continued societal interest in ethics and values, individuals are increasingly aware of the impact that acts of dishonesty have on themselves and their peers. A greater understanding of the role of professionals and their responsiveness to the consumer (whether defined as student, patient, client, or other) is essential when deliberating ethical problems to determine the most appropriate course of action.

Study Questions

1. What rights does FERPA protect and under what conditions may exceptions be made?

2. Why does FERPA affect so many institutions of higher education?

3. How do parental rights differ from a university's obligation to undergraduate and graduate students?

4. Describe the ethical and legal dilemmas of the department chair in this case. How do these differ from what you believe is morally "right" under the circumstances described? Are there a different set of dilemmas for the faculty, other students, or practitioners?

5. In considering academic dishonesty, what laws and ethical principles would you consider necessary to maintain a balance between an individual's right to privacy and the rights of the group as a whole?

Section 504 and Americans with Disabilities Act

CASE 1: A Student with Emotional Problems on Fieldwork Placement

CASE 2: A Student with a Physical Disability on Fieldwork Placement

with commentaries by **Barbara L. Kornblau, JD, OTR, FAOTA,** *and* **Penny Kyler, MA, OTR, FAOTA**

Key Terms

Antidiscrimination provisions of the ADA
Disability
Fieldwork site requirements
Impairment

Major life activities
Nondiscrimination
Public accommodation
Readily achievable

CASE 1: A Student with Emotional Problems on Fieldwork Placement

Eric, a level II fieldwork student, appears well qualified to handle the fieldwork experience during his placement interview with the fieldwork supervisor. One month later, however, when he begins to interact with the clients, his supervisor, Susan, notices that he is not always focused, is rather disorganized, and is not communicating well with the clients. Susan goes back to her interview notes and finds that Eric had a B+ average at school and has mentioned no problems with the academic portion of his occupational therapy program.

Over the next three weeks, there is no improvement in Eric's behavior. In fact, Susan notices additional problems with his memory and abstract thinking. In their weekly meeting, Susan tries to talk to Eric about his problems, but she gets nowhere. Finally, Susan calls the academic fieldwork coordinator at the school, who says that Eric has some emotional problems and that this information was not shared initially because Eric did not want the facility to know. The coordinator had encouraged Eric to share the information at the interview, but he chose not to do so.

The coordinator also added that the faculty had felt it was unlikely that Eric would successfully complete his level II fieldwork experiences, but that they had no reason to dismiss him from the program because he could manage the academic work adequately. What should Susan's course of action be?

CASE 2: A Student with a Physical Disability on Fieldwork Placement

Christine is interviewing for her level II fieldwork placement in physical dysfunction. She is an extremely able student, who has done very well in the academic portion of her program in occupational therapy. Christine has a partially atrophied left hand and forearm following childhood poliomyelitis and has been taught compensatory techniques throughout the curriculum for treatment activities requiring strength in both arms.

During the interview, Christine mentions her disability and states that it should not cause any difficulty during the affiliation and that she is confident she can manage any physical activities required of her. The interviewing supervisor, however, is not so sure and questions her about transferring clients. Christine is scheduled to work on a unit in which most clients have had cerebral vascular accidents or have paraplegia, and a great number of transfers will be needed. Although the supervisor can see that Christine is able to perform a transfer, he doubts her ability to do so repeatedly and is concerned for the safety of both the clients and Christine.

The supervisor wishes to move Christine's placement to a unit in which few transfers are needed, but Christine wants to gain experience with the types of clients on the unit originally suggested and feels she should be given the opportunity to try. A disagreement ensues and the student contacts the academic fieldwork coordinator at her school, asking for support in remaining on the original unit. What should be done?

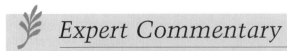

Expert Commentary

By Barbara L. Kornblau, JD, OTR, FAOTA

Purpose of the Americans with Disabilities Act

Box 3-1 *By the Law*

The ADA borrows from the 1973 Rehabilitation Act by defining an individual with a disability as a person who has a physical or mental **impairment** that substantially limits major life activities; has a record of such impairment; or is regarded as having such impairment. **Major life activities** means functions such as caring for one's self, performing manual tasks, walking, seeing, hearing, speaking, breathing, learning, and working.

Box 3-2 *Summary*

The goal of the ADA is to prevent discrimination against individuals with disabilities by extending the same civil rights protection guaranteed under the law to individuals on the basis of race, creed, sex, national origin, and religion. To promote its purpose, the ADA guarantees to millions of individuals with disabilities equal rights protection in the areas of employment, public accommodations, transportation, state and local governments, and telecommunications.

Congress passed the Americans with Disabilities Act (ADA) [Pub. L. No. 101–336 (1990) 42 U.S.C. 12101 et seq.] to provide persons with disabilities an opportunity to enter the world of work and to participate in the stream of independent living. The ADA is one of the most significant pieces of legislation to affect occupational therapy practice since the passage of the Education of the Handicapped Act, Pub. L. No. 94–142 (1975). It borrows from the 1973 Rehabilitation Act by defining an individual with a disability as a person who has a physical or mental impairment that substantially limits major life activities; has a record of such impairment; or is regarded as having such impairment. Major life activities means functions such as caring for one's self, performing manual tasks, walking, seeing, hearing, speaking, breathing, learning, and working (www.hhs.gov/ocr/ada.html, accessed 9/16/02) (Box 3-1).

The ADA was signed into law on July 26, 1990, broadly expanding opportunities for occupational therapy clients and occupational therapy practitioners with disabilities. Its goal is to prevent discrimination against individuals with disabilities by extending the same civil rights protection guaranteed under the law to individuals on the basis of race, creed, sex, national origin, and religion. To promote its purpose, the ADA guarantees to millions of individuals with disabilities equal rights protection in the areas of employment, public accommodations, transportation, state and local governments, and telecommunications (Box 3-2).

The ADA broadens the prior law, Section 504 of the Rehabilitation Act of 1973 (Section 504), Pub. L. No. 93–516 (1973), as amended (29 U.S.C. 794). Section 504 prohibits discrimination against persons with disabilities by entities that receive or benefit from federal funds. Section 504 excludes Veterans Administration and other federal government hospitals, which are subject to Section 501 of the Rehabilitation Act of 1973. Because almost every hospital and university or college in the United States receives or benefits from federal funds through some avenue, such as federally guaranteed student loans or research grants, these institutions fell under the antidiscrimination provisions of Section 504 before the passage of the ADA.

Box 3-3 *By the Law*

Antidiscrimination provisions of the ADA have been extended to all non–state government employers with 15 or more employees, to state and local government services, and to all places of public accommodations regardless of whether they receive federal funds.

In extending the antidiscrimination provisions of the ADA to all non–state government employers with 15 or more employees, to state and local government services, and to all places of public accommodations regardless of whether they receive federal funds (*Board of Trustees of the University of Alabama* v. *Garrett*, 2001) (Box 3-3). Congress also gave individuals with disabilities easier access to the judicial system. Although Section 504 places some limitations on individuals' access to the judicial system and their ability to recover monetary damages and other relief, the ADA allows a broader range of relief. Furthermore, the ADA allows direct access to the courts by individuals who face discrimination from places of public accommodation.

The ADA and Section 504 present interesting dilemmas to occupational therapy practitioners and occupational therapy students who are learning to deal appropriately in their own profession with individuals who have disabilities. This chapter focuses on two typical dilemmas faced by students, clinical supervisors, and academic educators because of the requirements of the ADA and Section 504.

Section 504 of the Rehabilitation Act

The occupational therapy profession recognizes the need for occupational therapy practitioners to keep abreast of current federal and state laws and regulations affecting the profession, such as the Standards of Practice for Occupational Therapy (American Occupational Therapy Association [AOTA], 1998a). Before analyzing an ethical dilemma involving discrimination on the basis of disability in a fieldwork setting, one must understand the basic concepts of the relevant laws—Section 504 and the ADA.

Section 504, the precursor to the ADA, simply states:

> No otherwise qualified handicapped individual in the United States . . . shall, solely by reason of his handicap, be excluded from

participation in, be denied the benefits of, or be subjected to discrimination under any program or activity receiving Federal financial assistance or under any program or activity conducted by any Executive agency or by the United States Post Office.

(29 U.S.C. 794)

"Handicap" in Section 504 included three definitions similar to those found for "disability" in the ADA. Handicap is defined as one who:

"Has a physical or mental impairment that substantially limits one or more of the major life activities"

"Has a record of such impairment"

"Is regarded as having a handicap"

[28 C.F.R. section 41.31(a) (b)]

Department of Justice regulations defined "qualified handicapped person" with respect to services as "a person who meets the essential eligibility requirements for the receipt of such services" (28 C.F.R. section 41.32). According to the U.S. Department of Education, for purposes of postsecondary education services, "a qualified handicapped person is an individual with handicap(s) who meets the academic and technical standards requisite to admission or participation in the recipient's education program or activity" (U.S. Department of Education, 1989). In *Southeastern Community College* v. *Davis*, 442 U.S. 2361 (1979), the U.S. Supreme Court defined "an otherwise qualified person" under Section 504 as one who is able to meet all of a program's requirements in spite of his handicap." Although Section 504 originally referred to individuals with disabilities as "handicapped," the law has been amended because this term is no longer acceptable. Its further use in this chapter will be substituted with the phrase "individual with a disability."

The term "program or activity" includes (1) state and local government agencies and entities that receive federal funds; (2) entire colleges, universities, or school systems; and (3) corporations or other private organizations that are engaged in providing education, health care, housing, social services, parks and recreation, or entities that receive federal financial assistance as a whole [Civil Rights Restoration Act, Pub. L. No. 100–259 (1988)]. Hospitals and other healthcare clinics serving as fieldwork sites thus fall subject to Section 504's requirements because at a minimum, they receive federal funding in the form of Medicare, Medicaid, TRI-CARE/CHAMPUS, or federal workers' compensation medical benefit payments. Most colleges and universities receive or benefit from federal funds through the federally guaranteed student loan programs, grants, and other sources.

Box 3-4 *By the Law*

Section 504 requires postsecondary institutions to operate in a nondiscriminatory manner in recruitment, admission, academic programs, research, occupational training, housing, counseling, and other areas. Postsecondary institutions cannot contract with fieldwork sites whose employees discriminate against students with disabilities.

Section 504 requires postsecondary institutions to operate in a nondiscriminatory manner in recruitment, admission, academic programs, research, occupational training, housing, counseling, and other areas. Postsecondary institutions cannot contract with fieldwork sites whose employees discriminate against students with disabilities (Box 3-4).

According to Section 504, students with disabilities must be given an equal opportunity to participate in and benefit from all postsecondary education programs and activities, including education programs and activities not operated wholly by the school (U.S. Department of Education, 1989). All programs must be offered in the most integrated setting possible. Section 504 requires that academic requirements be modified on a case-by-case basis to afford qualified students with disabilities an equal opportunity; however, academic requirements, which federal funds recipients demonstrate are essential, will not be regarded as discriminatory (U.S. Department of Education, 1989).

Section 504 prohibits recipients or those who benefit from federal funds from imposing rules on students with disabilities that limit their participation. Finally, students with disabilities must be given the opportunity to participate in any course, any course of study, or any other part of the education program or activity offered by a recipient of federal funds.

The Americans with Disabilities Act

Titles I and II

The ADA is the other relevant law that must be examined in relation to fieldwork issues. Title I, the Employment Provisions, prohibits non–state government employers with 15 or more employees from discriminating against employees and applicants with disabilities (29 C.F.R. section 1630). Title II, State and Local Government Services, prohibits state and local government agencies such as counties and municipalities from discriminating against individuals with disabilities in the provision of services, other than employment by a state government. Title II requires state and local government hospitals and clinics to abide by numerous antidiscrimination rules that are similar to Title III (28 C.F.R. section 35.101 et seq.). Title III, the public accommodations section, prohibits places of public accommodations that are not government owned from discriminating against individuals with disabilities (28 C.F.R. 36 section 101 et seq.).

If the issues in this chapter dealt with matters of employment other than employment with a state entity, Title I would govern these ethical dilemmas. If the fieldwork settings in these ethical dilemmas involved state-run or county-run hospitals or clinics, Title II would govern the hypothetical scenarios. If the fieldwork sites in the case scenarios took place in a federal government facility such as a Veterans Administration hospital, the ADA would not apply at all because the federal government is exempt from the ADA. Federal institutions are subject to the requirements of Section 501 of the Rehabilitation Act of 1973, which has similar requirements to those of Section 504 and the ADA. Because the ethical dilemmas in this chapter deal with fieldwork issues not involving employment or federal, state, or local government run facilities, Title III of the ADA, the Public Accommodations Provision, governs these situations.

Title III

Title III, which took effect on January 26, 1992, promotes inclusion of individuals with disabilities in all programs offered by places of public accommodations. Title III's main purpose is to allow access to goods, programs, services, facilities, and advantages offered at a place of public accommodation (28 C.F.R. Part 36). The regulations require places of public accommodations, including but not limited to retail establishments, movie theaters, hospitals, hotels, doctors' offices, restaurants, and schools, to make changes that are "readily achievable" to provide access to the goods, programs, services, facilities, and advantages that they offer (28 C.F.R. section 36.104). Readily achievable is defined as changes that are easily accomplishable and able to be carried out without much difficulty or expense (28 C.F.R. section 36.304) (Box 3-5).

Box 3-5 *By the Law*

Title III of the ADA regulations requires places of **public accommodations,** including but not limited to retail establishments, movie theaters, hospitals, hotels, doctors' offices, restaurants, and schools, to make changes that are "readily achievable" to provide access to the goods, programs, services, facilities, and advantages that they offer. **Readily achievable** is defined as changes that are easily accomplishable and able to be carried out without much difficulty or expense.

Unfortunately, many people often view the scope of Title III as physical or architectural accessibility guidelines only; however, Title III is concerned with more than mere physical access to a building. Title III requires places of public accommodation to give individuals with disabilities equal opportunity to participate in and benefit from all programs, goods, services, programs, facilities, and advantages provided by the place of public accommodation in the most integrated setting appropriate (28 C.F.R. sections 36.202, 36.203).

Definition of Disability

Like Section 504, the ADA gives three definitions for the term "disability." First, **disability** is defined as a physical or mental impairment that substantially limits one or more of the individual's major life activities (28 C.F.R. section 36.104). Physical or mental impairment includes any physiological disorder or condition, cosmetic disfigurement, or anatomical loss affecting one or more of the following body systems: neurological, musculoskeletal, special sense organs, respiratory (including speech organs), cardiovascular, reproductive, digestive, genitourinary, hemic and lymphatic, skin, and endocrine. Mental impairments include mental or psychological disorders such as mental retardation, organic brain syndrome, emotional or mental illness, and specific learning disabilities (28 C.F.R. section 36.104).

"Major life activities" include functions such as caring for oneself, performing manual tasks, walking, seeing, hearing, speaking, breathing, learning, and working (28 C.F.R. section 36.104). An "impairment" substantially interferes with a major life activity when these activities are restricted regarding the conditions, manner, or duration under which the individual can perform in comparison to most people (U.S. Department of Justice, 1992, section III-2.4000; the Tech Manual). In interpreting major life activities in an employment context, the U.S. Supreme Court provided some additional guidance for those who claim to be substantially limited in the specific major life activity of "performing manual tasks." Stressing the extreme nature and severity inherent in the words "substantially limiting," the Court stated that "an individual must have an impairment that prevents or severely restricts the individual from doing activities that are of central importance to most people's daily lives" (*Toyota Motor Mfg., Kentucky, Inc.* v. *Williams,* 2002). The Courts will continue to hear challenges to the ADA and may make other changes in its interpretation of this and other sections of the ADA over time.

The second definition of disability is physical or mental impairment that substantially limits one or more of the individual's major life activities and includes individuals with a record of such impairments (28 C.F.R. section 36.104). For example, the individual who has cancer now in remission, a history of back surgery to remedy a back impairment, or a history of mental or emotional illness or drug addiction would find protection under this definition.

The third definition of disability encompasses individuals who are regarded as having a disability whether they have the impairment or not (Tech Manual section III 2.1000; 28 C.F.R. section 36.104). These individuals may not in fact have a disability; however, they are protected by the ADA because others perceive them as having a disability and treat them differently based on that perception. For example, an individual who has a severe facial scar or who is thought to have acquired immunodeficiency syndrome (AIDS) based on a rumor would find protection under the third definition.

Principles for Nondiscrimination and Their Implementation

Title III of the ADA enumerates three broad principles for nondiscrimination: (1) equal opportunity to participate, (2) equal opportunity to benefit, and (3) equal opportunity to receive benefits in the most integrated setting appropriate (Tech Manual III-3.1000) (Box 3-6).

To implement these principles, Title III sets forth several rules that places of public accommodations must follow to govern their conduct. These rules apply to most fieldwork settings because most hospitals, clinics, colleges, and universities are places of public accommodations.

Eligibility Criteria

One of the most significant rules prevents fieldwork sites, as places of public accommodations, from imposing eligibility criteria that screen out persons with disabilities unless the criteria are necessary for the provision of the goods, programs, services, privileges, advantages, or accommodations (28 C.F.R. 36.301). Fieldwork sites must also integrate students with disabilities to the maximum extent appropriate (Tech Manual section III-3.4000). In other words, a fieldwork site could not force a student into a separate or special program unless the student's disability required a separate program. In providing goods and services, a public accommodation may not use eligibility requirements that exclude or segregate individuals with disabilities, unless the requirements are necessary for the operation of the public accommodation (Box 3-7).

Policy Modifications

Fieldwork sites must make reasonable modifications to their policies, practices, and procedures to accommodate persons with disabilities (28

C.F.R. section 36.302). For example, this may include allowing a field-work student to bring a service dog to work each day, although dogs are not normally allowed in the clinic. Public accommodations are not required to make modifications that would fundamentally alter the nature of the services provided (28 C.F.R. section 36.302). For example, if a student came to the fieldwork site with a disability that caused her to be light sensitive, it would not be a reasonable accommodation to lower the lights because this would create a safety hazard for most of the elderly clients in the clinic.

Auxiliary Aides and Services

Fieldwork sites are also required to provide auxiliary aides and services to ensure effective communication with the student with a disability [28 C.F.R. section 36.303 (c)]. "Auxiliary aids and services" include what occupational therapy practitioners call adaptive equipment and also may include qualified interpreters, note-takers, telecommunications devices for the deaf, videotext displays, volume-control telephones, closed-captioned or open-captioned videotapes, or materials in Braille (28 C.F.R. section 36.303). For example, a fieldwork site might have to have someone take notes for a student with a learning disability at an in-service training. Extra charges may not be imposed on individuals with disabilities to cover the costs of measures necessary to ensure nondiscriminatory treatment, such as removing barriers or providing sign language interpreters; however, there is no requirement to provide aids to students such as individually prescribed wheelchairs or glasses, or to provide personal services such as assistance with toileting (28 C.F.R. section 36.306).

Architectural and Structural Barriers

Fieldwork sites must remove architectural or other structural barriers in existing facilities to the extent that such steps are "readily achievable." "Readily achievable" means easily accomplishable and able to be carried out without much difficulty or expense (28 C.F.R. section 36.104). If barrier removal is not readily achievable, the fieldwork site must make its goods, services, programs, facilities, and advantages available by alternative methods or by providing auxiliary aides (28 C.F.R. section 36.305). For example, a fieldwork site would be required to install a ramp to allow access for an affiliating student in a wheelchair to the hand clinic. If installing a ramp is not readily achievable, the clinic would be required to seek alternatives such as moving the student's clients and equipment to an accessible location; however, accommodations do not have to be provided if the accommodations impose an undue burden or require significant difficulty or expense to provide (28 C.F.R. section 36.104).

Safety Requirements

Safety requirements may be imposed only if necessary for the safe operation of a place of public accommodation (28 C.F.R. section 36.208). They must be based on actual risks and not on mere speculation, stereotypes, or generalizations about individuals with disabilities. For example, a clinical supervisor could not refuse a placement to a fieldwork student with epilepsy because he is worried that the student might have a seizure and injure clients. This would be based on speculation and generalizations.

Outside Contracts

Finally, Title III prohibits places of public accommodation from contracting with others who perpetuate discriminatory acts. Thus an occupational therapy program at a college or university, as a place of public accommodation, could not contract with a fieldwork site that discriminates against students with disabilities.

Relationship of Ethics to Law

Before analyzing ethical dilemmas that involve legal issues, the occupational therapy practitioner must look at the relationship of ethics to law. Many sources of rules and regulations govern the conduct of occupational therapy practitioners. These sources include state licensure laws, malpractice standards, state and federal criminal or civil statutes, and case law. Thus there are several standards with which the occupational therapy practitioner's conduct will be compared. There are also several non–legally binding documents that are guides to practice and reflect the norms within the occupational therapy community. These documents including the AOTA Code of Ethics, Guidelines to the Occupational Therapy Code of Ethics, Standards of Practice for Occupational Therapy, and The Core Values and Attitudes of Occupational Therapy Practice.

The occupational therapy practitioner must look at the various sources to determine whether his or her conduct is reconcilable. After examining the considerations from all sources, the practitioner may be faced with conflicts. Practitioners may find that their actions violate one of these systems or standards but not another. Therefore, the behavior may subject the participants to a wide range of sanctions. For example, an action may be repugnant, such as requiring all noninsured clients to pay cash up front before treatment, but may not be civilly actionable or malpractice. On the other hand, a practitioner's conduct may be legal, ethical, and not a violation of a state licensure law, but civilly actionable, such as violating a noncompete clause of a contract. The occupational therapy practitioner faces different risks or sanctions depending on his or her choice of action.

Because this chapter focuses on fieldwork situations and the ADA, the academic fieldwork coordinator and clinical supervisor will want to choose a course of action that is both legal and ethical, and that complies with the Standards of Practice for Occupational Therapy and the AOTA Code of Ethics. The wrong choice could lead to an ADA Title III lawsuit filed against either the school or the fieldwork site, or an investigation by the Department of Justice.

Ethical Analysis

The ADA will present many ethical dilemmas to occupational therapists in practice, management, and fieldwork supervision situations. Ethical dilemmas do not present themselves in prepackaged form, labeled with a warning. Ethical dilemmas arise as an integral part of practice. Knowing an isolated list of ethics rules and government regulations does little good for the practitioner. Rather, the practitioner must know how to identify, analyze, and respond to potentially arduous situations that may involve ethical and legal issues.

The ethical dilemmas in this chapter, involving the ADA and Section 504 in a fieldwork setting, are examples of such challenging situations. Several systems of ethical analysis have been developed to guide the professional in resolving the conflict that arises when one faces an ethical dilemma. Hansen and Kyler-Hutchison (1992) developed a method of analyzing ethical dilemmas in occupational therapy based on the work of Aroskar and associates. This system of analysis requires that one answer the following questions:

1. Who are the players?
2. What other facts or information do you need?
3. What actions might be taken?
4. What are the consequences of each action ethically, medically, or legally?

Based on the answers to these questions, one must then "choose an action and defend it" (p. 628). In everyday practice, I often employ the Hansen and Kyler method of analysis combined with a variation of the Rotary International four-way test (Rotary International, 1990) to analyze actions chosen in response to ethical dilemmas. The Rotary four-way test asks the following questions:

1. Is it the truth?
2. Is it fair to all concerned?
3. Will it build goodwill and better friendships?
4. Will it be beneficial to all concerned?

Here, a variation adds to the first question "And/or is it legal?" Finally, any ethical analysis of an ADA issue must include an examination of the AOTA Code of Ethics (2000a) and the Standards of Practice for Occupational Therapy (1998a), as well as the applicable and relevant sections of the ADA.

The ADA directly affects the way students, clinical supervisors, and fieldwork coordinators interact. The cases presented at the beginning of the chapter will be used to explore these interactions.

Case 1: A Student with Emotional Problems on Fieldwork Placement

Before analyzing what action to take in the case of Eric, the student with emotional problems on a fieldwork placement, the action that has already occurred must be analyzed. Under the ADA, to be entitled to a reasonable accommodation, the individual must have a disability and must identify the need for an accommodation. The obligation of a place of public accommodation to make reasonable accommodations for an individual arises only when it has knowledge that this person is an individual with a disability in need of accommodation. In other words, a hospital or clinic, as a place of public accommodation, has no obligation to accommodate a person unless it knows that the person needs an accommodation. The person is not required to identify himself or herself as an individual with a disability unless he or she needs to be reasonably accommodated.

In this ethical dilemma, Eric has chosen not to identify himself as an individual with a disability to Susan, his fieldwork supervisor. This, in turn, poses an interesting dilemma for the academic fieldwork coordinator. By telling Susan about Eric's emotional problems, she has violated both Section 504 of the Rehabilitation Act and the Family Educational Rights and Privacy Act (FERPA). Section 504 requires that information acquired about an individual's disability be kept confidential. FERPA requires educational institutions to keep all educational records confidential unless they have been specifically permitted by the student to release the information. Because Eric did not want the facility to know about his emotional problems and because he did not give his permission to release the information, the academic fieldwork coordinator violated the law by breaching his confidentiality.

This breach of confidentiality under Section 504 and FERPA violates the Standards of Practice for Occupational Therapy Standard I, Professional Standing and Responsibility, Section 2, which states: "An occupational therapy practitioner delivers occupational therapy services in accordance with AOTA's standards and policies. The nature and scope of occupational therapy services provided must be in accordance with laws and regulations." In addition, by violating Section 504 and FERPA, the academic fieldwork coordinator violates the AOTA Code of Ethics, Principle 5, Compliance with Laws and Regulations. This principle states: "Occupational therapy personnel shall comply with laws and Association policies guiding the profession of occupational therapy." Therefore, the academic fieldwork coordinator breached the AOTA

Standards of Practice and Code of Ethics by failing to keep Eric's information confidential.

The academic fieldwork coordinator has an obligation to be aware of current laws that affect practice. She should have been aware of her obligation to keep the disclosed information confidential. The Standards of Practice for Occupational Therapy, Standard I, Professional Standing states: "An occupational therapy practitioner maintains current knowledge of legislative, political, social, cultural, and reimbursement issues that affect clients and the practice of occupational therapy."

The academic fieldwork coordinator also had an obligation to inform Susan of her obligation to comply with the ADA. The AOTA Code of Ethics, Principle 3, Compliance with Laws and Regulations, states: "Occupational therapy practitioners shall remain abreast of revisions in those laws and Association policies that apply to the profession of occupational therapy and shall inform employers, employees, and colleagues of those changes." The academic fieldwork coordinator had an obligation under the Standards of Practice to know about the ADA and its effect on students. Furthermore, she had an obligation to inform the fieldwork supervisor of the ADA and its effect on students. The academic fieldwork coordinator failed to meet these obligations, and her actions are unethical and a violation of the ADA.

Because the academic fieldwork coordinator divulged confidential information about Eric's emotional problems to Susan, Susan is now on notice that Eric may be an individual with a disability. Whether his emotional problems constitute a mental impairment according to the ADA, it seems as if he is being regarded by the faculty as having a mental impairment in the form of an "emotional illness." According to the academic fieldwork coordinator, the faculty sees Eric's emotional problems as substantially limiting his ability to successfully complete his level II fieldwork placement. Therefore, Eric may fit the category of an individual with the third definition of disability—an individual who is regarded as having a disability. If Eric does not have a disability and is not regarded as having a disability, he is not entitled to any reasonable accommodation.

What Actions Can Susan Take?

First, Susan can focus on whether Eric is an individual with a disability, but with these particular facts, this is not a black-or-white issue. It would be helpful to know additional facts about the extent of Eric's disability. Without these facts, Susan faces two alternatives. First, she can proceed as if Eric were an individual with a disability because more than likely he will fit within the ADA's third definition. Alternately, pursuant to Section 504 and the ADA, Susan may ask Eric directly, on a confidential basis, whether he is an individual with a disability. This is intended to determine whether Eric requires accommodations for his disability.

If Susan makes a direct inquiry about Eric's disability and he fails to admit that he is an individual with a disability, Susan is still on notice that the faculty regards him as having a substantially limiting emotional impairment. With this knowledge, if Susan does not treat Eric as an individual with a disability, she may subject her employer to an ADA Title III federal lawsuit and/or an investigation by the U.S. Department of Justice. The safest alternative is to treat Eric as if he is an individual with a disability.

After Susan receives notice that Eric is an individual with a disability, the obligation to reasonably accommodate Eric's disability may arise. If Susan fails to attempt to accommodate Eric's disability, her facility may face charges of discrimination. Initially, Susan should explain to Eric that he is not performing as expected or required to successfully complete fieldwork. She should explain her legal obligation to accommodate an individual with a disability and ask Eric if he requires accommodations. As the courts have interpreted the ADA, however, most agree that the obligation to accommodate only arises after the individual with a disability expressly discloses his or her disability and makes a specific request for a specific accommodation (*Morisky* v. *Broward County*, 1996; *Gaston* v. *Belhingrath Garden & Home, Inc.*, 1999).

Susan may be able to develop some accommodations for Eric in concert with him, using their combined occupational therapy knowledge. If Eric informs Susan that he has an emotional disability and is under the care of a mental health professional, with Eric's consent that professional also may be consulted for assistance with developing reasonable accommodations to enable Eric to successfully complete the affiliation.

For example, perhaps Eric's memory problems can be accommodated by carrying a personal digital assistant (PDA) such as a palm pilot or pocket notepad for making frequent notes about items he needs to remember. To address Eric's problem with disorganization, he may need supervision on how to better organize and schedule his day or use the PDA to outline his schedule while incorporating built-in alarm features. If Eric is going through a particular emotional setback, a leave from the fieldwork placement until his mental health professional indicates he is fit to return might reasonably accommodate him.

There may not be any reasonable accommodations to allow Eric to successfully complete his affiliation. If the accommodations fail to enable him to complete the affiliation despite being given an equal opportunity to participate in and benefit from the affiliation program at this fieldwork site, Eric cannot meet the essential academic requirements. He may not be an otherwise qualified individual if he cannot meet all of the program's requirements despite his disability. Therefore, after legitimate but unsuccessful attempts to accommodate Eric's disability, Susan can terminate his fieldwork or give him a failing grade, as she would do with any nondisabled student. As long as Susan made a good faith attempt to reasonably accommodate Eric's disability, her actions in terminating him or failing him would be legal and ethical.

If Eric were not able to complete the affiliation with reasonable accommodations, the school would not be required to eliminate or "water down" his affiliation. Doing so would significantly lower the standards for Eric and bring into question other occupational therapy students' degree requirements and training. According to the U.S. Supreme Court, in *Southeastern Community College* v. *Davis*, 442 U.S. 2361 (1979), Section 504 imposes no duty on educational institutions to lower or to make substantial modifications to standards to accommodate individuals with disabilities, especially where institutions train persons to render professional services. To be fair to all parties concerned, Susan and the occupational therapy program at the college must maintain the same standards for all students.

Case 2: A Student with a Physical Disability on Fieldwork Placement

In the second case, concerning a student with a physical disability, the first step is to look at the action already taken. As already reviewed in the overview of Title III of the ADA, a fieldwork site may not use eligibility requirements that exclude or segregate individuals with disabilities, unless the requirements are "necessary" for its operation. According to the facts presented, the interviewing supervisor doubts Christine's ability to perform repeated transfers and has a concern about client safety. Because of these concerns, the supervisor wishes to segregate Christine on another unit.

What is the Basis for the Supervisor's Concern?

If the supervisor is basing his decision on the mere fact that Christine has a partially atrophied left hand and forearm and therefore shouldn't be transferring clients, he sounds the call of discrimination. His refusal is only legitimate if not allowing Christine to transfer clients is necessary for the safe operation of the unit. Before the supervisor can make the decision to exclude Christine from a unit that requires extensive transfers, he must be prepared to show that Christine poses a "direct threat" to clients. Title III seeks to protect individuals with disabilities from discrimination based on prejudice, stereotypes, or unfounded fear, while giving appropriate weight to legitimate concerns, such as the need to avoid exposing others to significant health and safety risks.

According to the Title III Technical Assistance Manual, "a public accommodation may exclude an individual with a disability from participation in an activity, if that individual's participation would result in a direct threat to the health or safety of others" (Tech Manual section III-3.8000). To support the direct threat assertion, the supervisor must determine that Christine poses a significant risk to others that cannot be eliminated or reduced to an acceptable level by reasonably modifying the clinic's policies, practices, or procedures, or by providing appropriate auxiliary aides or services.

The determination of whether Christine poses a direct threat to the health or safety of the clients may not be based on generalizations or stereotypes about the effects of her particular disability. It must be based on an individual assessment that considers the particular activity— transfers—and Christine's actual abilities (Tech Manual section III-3.8000, 28 C.F.R. section 36.208). The individualized assessment must be based on reasonable judgment that relies on current medical evidence, or on the best available objective evidence, to determine the following criteria:

1. The nature, duration, and severity of the risk
2. The probability that the potential injury will actually occur
3. Whether reasonable modifications of policies, practices, or procedures will mitigate or eliminate the risk (Tech Manual section III-3.8000)

In the employment context, the Equal Employment Opportunity Commission (EEOC), the administrative agency that enforces Title I of the ADA, changed its regulations to add activities that directly threaten one's *own* health and safety in addition to those causing a direct threat to the health or safety of others (29 CFR section 1630.15(b)(2), 2001). The U.S. Supreme Court upheld this regulation in *Chevron U.S.A. Inc.* v. *Echazabal,* 2002. Although this case comes from the employment arena, because fieldwork is so similar to a worklike setting, the courts would probably use a similar standard if Christine's fieldwork imposed a direct threat to her.

When viewing the safety issues, the supervisor obviously failed to analyze the situation completely according to the ADA mandates. After all, Christine had demonstrated proper performance of transfers throughout her educational program. The supervisor's concerns about repeated transfers appear to be unfounded if one analyzes the elements of the required individualized assessment as mandated by the ADA. Direct threat from placing Christine in the high-number-of-transfers unit poses only a speculative risk and certainly falls short of the ADA requisite direct threat requirement. Christine properly performs the transfers; therefore the nature, duration, and severity of the risk of harming a client during a transfer is minimal and not more than with any other student. Furthermore, the probability that harm will occur is uncertain. The supervisor only doubts Christine's ability to transfer repeatedly, which indicates a low probability and uncertainty that potential harm will occur at all.

Finally, even if Christine's physical disability posed a higher risk to the clients, reasonable accommodations could greatly reduce or eliminate the risk. For example, suppose fatigue prevented Christine from performing transfers in the afternoon. It would probably be reasonable to have other staff members—occupational therapists and physical therapists as well as aides and transporters—assist Christine with the afternoon transfers. Occupational and physical therapy clinic staff members, aides, transporters, and nurses often assist pregnant therapists with transfers when such assistance is needed. Accommodating Christine in this manner would be no different.

In most cases, transferring clients is not an essential job function for an occupational therapy practitioner. Title I of the ADA (employment) and its implementing regulations define "essential functions" of the job as the fundamental job duties of the position the person desires or holds [29 C.F.R. section 1630.2(n)]. Essential functions are the basic job duties that an employee must be able to perform, with or without reasonable accommodation.

Factors to consider in determining whether a function is essential include the following:

▶ Whether the reason the position exists is to perform that function

▶ The number of other employees who are available to perform the function or among whom the performance of the functions can be distributed

▶ The degree of expertise or skill required to perform the function [29 CFR section 1630.2(n)(2), Equal Employment Opportunity Commission, 1992 section 2.3]

Occupational therapy positions do not exist to transfer clients. Other professionals and staff members in a clinic are also trained to perform transfers. In most situations, especially where students require supervision, other staff members could assist with the transfers if they became a problem for Christine.

Finally, transferring clients does not take special expertise possessed only by an occupational therapy practitioner. Possessing the knowledge of how to do transfers is the essential function. Christine could describe how the transfer is done and instruct someone else to assist her by actually performing the proper transfer.

No one has alleged that Christine imposes a direct threat to her own health and safety. Christine does not pose a direct threat to her clients because she has demonstrated to her supervisor that she is able to safely perform transfers. Even if she were not able to consistently do this task, she could be accommodated by having others assist her, thereby eliminating any risk she might pose to her clients.

What Actions Should Be Taken?

According to the Standards of Practice for Occupational Therapy and the AOTA Code of Ethics, the fieldwork supervisor has an obligation to maintain current knowledge of legislative and political issues affecting occupational therapy. The supervisor has a further obligation to comply with laws and Association policies guiding the profession of occupational therapy. To segregate Christine violates Section 504, the ADA, and possibly state law. Furthermore, this action falls below the Standards of Practice and violates the AOTA Code of Ethics. Thus segregation of this kind is both illegal and unethical.

The academic fieldwork coordinator has an obligation, according to the Standards of Practice and the AOTA Code of Ethics, to be knowledgeable about the ADA and to inform the clinical supervisor of the ADA's requirements. The academic fieldwork coordinator should support Christine and explain to the clinical supervisor that segregating Christine at this time is discriminatory. Christine has been taught compensatory techniques for the transfers and has demonstrated her competency and skill. The analysis of the direct threat provisions shows that Christine may be accommodated to enable her to stay on the unit she prefers and to safely transfer clients. Although Christine may need assistance at some time in the future, she does not show that she poses a significant risk to her clients.

The academic fieldwork coordinator should encourage the clinical supervisor to place Christine on the unit as originally planned because she qualifies for the placement. The coordinator should inform the clinical supervisor that to segregate Christine from clients requiring transfers is discriminatory and violates Section 504 and Title III of the ADA. This action may subject the fieldwork site to an investigation by the U.S. Department of Justice or a lawsuit. The academic fieldwork coordinator should encourage the supervisor to comply with the ADA and not to treat Christine any differently from any other affiliating student. The clinical supervisor should assure Christine that neither she nor any other staff members will penalize her for asking for assistance with transfers, if she finds herself in need of assistance. The supervisor should encourage Christine to ask for assistance when needed.

Christine is a wonderful role model for her clients. She has overcome some of the same impairments her clients now face. The academic fieldwork coordinator could try this line of reasoning with the supervisor. If all else fails, the coordinator should remind the supervisor that the occupational therapy program cannot continue to contract with the clinic if it perpetuates discrimination against its students.

Conclusion

Occupational therapy has witnessed the passage of numerous laws and regulations that have affected practice: Medicare, the Omnibus Budget Reconciliation Act (OBRA), licensure, Pub. L. No 94-142, and diagnostic related groups (DRGs), to name a few. The ADA is merely another regulation with which the profession must learn to cope. Although change often momentarily steers an individual from his or her chosen path, the ADA will soon become a familiar guidepost. Occupational therapy practitioners will adapt to meet the ADA's challenge to provide fieldwork students with a fair, ethical, and legal chance to succeed along the path to their goal of entering the profession.

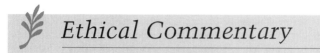

Ethical Commentary

By Penny Kyler, MA, OTR, FAOTA

Cases 1 and 2: Students with a Disability on Fieldwork Placements

In general, occupational therapists want people to have successful experiences. Usually, that success is built on a collaborative relationship between the therapist and the client, the student, or the family. According to AOTA, students with disabilities have the right to be seen first as qualified, capable students and second as students who have disabilities. According to recent government information, more than 54 million Americans have disabilities, a full 20 percent of the U.S. population. Almost half of these individuals have a severe disability, affecting their ability to see, hear, walk, or perform other basic functions of life. In addition, more than 25 million family caregivers and millions more provide aid and assistance to people with disabilities (www.whitehouse.gov/news/freedominitiative/freedominitiative.html, accessed September 18, 2002).

The case scenarios of Eric and Christine, although different, describe the important relationship between a student and a fieldwork supervisor. Eric's case illustrates how nondisclosure can be a problem, and Christine's case illustrates how her need to succeed is impeded by her supervisor.

Who Are the Players?

The players are Eric, Christine, their fieldwork supervisors, the academic fieldwork coordinator, hospital and university attorneys, clients, administrators at the fieldwork site, and the university. Are there any others?

What Other Information Is Needed?

How much does the fieldwork supervisor know about the ADA? What are Eric's strengths and weaknesses regarding his therapeutic use of self, client assessment skills, and clinical reasoning skills? How has the supervisor attempted to organize Eric? What types of conversations have occurred? Is there a rapport and trust between therapist and student? Is it a fast-paced environment?

Regarding Christine, one might ask: What compensation techniques has she been taught before the fieldwork? What is the extent of her muscle strength and coordination? To what other client population could she be assigned? As an occupational therapist, what type of population does she wish to work with in the future?

For both students, what has transpired between the fieldwork supervisor and the academic fieldwork coordinator? Do either of these students have mentors or peers with whom they can discuss their concerns and frustrations before talking with their fieldwork supervisor? What other information would you like to have before making a decision about this case?

Rights and Duties of the Players

In thinking about the case, consider how American society has sometimes devalued individuals with disabilities. In Holmes and Purdy's *Feminist Perspectives in Medical Ethics*, Susan Wendell (1992) notes that there is an important issue to consider regarding the high value Americans place on independence versus gaining help from others. This concept is important because independence and fitness are still esteemed in this masculine and patriarchal culture. Two questions to consider that often go unasked are: What are the positives that an individual with disabilities brings to the mix? What types of reciprocity can be developed?

In the case scenarios, the rights and duties of the student, the fieldwork supervisor, and the academic fieldwork coordinator need to be distinguished. These rights and duties are clearly articulated in the Occupational Therapy Code of Ethics and the Guidelines to the Occupational Therapy Code of Ethics. Additional guidelines and information may also be available from the AOTA's Commission on Education.

Rights and Duties of the Student

One can assume that Eric and Christine have paid to do their fieldwork; therefore, the school has an obligation to provide them with a learning experience. Both have to fulfill certain performance requirements to receive a passing grade. As students, their duties consist of following the protocols of the facility in which they are doing their fieldwork, discussing actions with the supervisor before implementing them, and demonstrating a willingness to learn. They also have an obligation to be able to clearly discuss the rationale behind their clinical reasoning and the selection of the activity or modality for treatment. Furthermore, students have duties to those clients to whom they are assigned and should frankly and honestly consider their skill sets, liability issues, and future professional goals before working with these clients. In considering the issues, students have to be able to look beyond themselves and their immediate needs to the more global needs of the community—a community composed of the therapists who are student supervisors, the staff at the facility, and the clients they will be treating.

Rights and Duties of the Fieldwork Supervisor

Fieldwork supervisors have duties to their employer and their clients. They also have obligations to the academic institution that sends the students. They have duties to provide good, safe, and proficient client care as well as to follow all applicable guidelines, laws, and regulations that govern the practice of occupational therapy. In addition to these concrete duties, fieldwork supervisors by virtue of being occupational therapists have a duty to abide by the Occupational Therapy Code of Ethics and to treat their colleagues with respect. Inherent in this concept of respect are such things as using a positive approach and demonstrating concern for the dignity and respect of the individual, in this case the students. If needed, they may be able to accomplish this show of respect by providing an environment that allows students the time and privacy to share personal information.

Rights and Duties of the Academic Fieldwork Coordinator

The academic fieldwork coordinator has a duty to the students to facilitate learning experiences. She also has a duty to her employer (the academic institution) and to the clients to whom students will be assigned. The academic faculty in many ways become the protector of the public because they pass or fail students in their academic programs and allow them to move forward to fieldwork.

The academic fieldwork coordinator has a duty to evaluate problems that may arise between the student and the fieldwork supervisor and to facilitate resolutions in areas of dispute. She also has a duty to keep abreast of current issues and concerns regarding individuals with disabilities and the profession of occupational therapy.

Client Needs

To what extent should the student's learning experience infringe on safe client care? The fieldwork supervisor in the case scenarios is struggling with this issue. The ADA specifically prohibits discrimination against an individual identified with a disabling condition, but Eric and Christine are not being denied an opportunity to participate in the fieldwork experience. Eric is being asked to clarify and justify his communication issues, and Christine is being asked to move to another area that does not necessitate her repeatedly transferring clients. Eric has not yet discussed his disability with the fieldwork supervisor, whereas Christine feels that she should be given the opportunity to succeed on a unit for clients with cerebral vascular accidents and paraplegia, where many transfers would be needed.

What Actions May Be Taken and What Are the Possible Consequences?

Actions that may be taken and the possible consequences to Eric have been thoroughly discussed by Ms. Kornblau. In both cases, the therapists involved should rationally evaluate their choices by blending integrity and prudence. They should consider occupational therapy's core value of dignity, which focuses on the inherent worth and uniqueness of each individual. Both of these students may or may not become excellent occupational therapy practitioners. In the meantime, their supervisors should consider their own actions in light of the Core Values and Attitudes (AOTA, 1993a) to mitigate against unnecessary, real, or imagined discrimination. In addition, they may wish to review Section 2 of the Guidelines to the Occupational Therapy Code of Ethics (1998b) concerning communication and take note that all practitioners should be honest in gathering and giving fact-based information.

Regarding Christine, two possible courses of action to safeguard clients' needs would be (1) to protect the clients from harm by not allowing Christine to do the transfers or (2) to engage the clients in decision making before treatment. I have chosen to present arguments in favor of the latter action.

Following this course of action, all clients would be told when they were being treated by students (not solely Christine) and would be invited to participate in their treatment process by deciding whether they wish to have a student or a therapist assist with their transfers. With any new client, Christine (and the other students) would explain her student status and ask clients if they had an objection to her assisting in their transfers. It is possible that some clients would be more receptive to working with Christine because she had mastered compensation techniques that might prove beneficial to clients. Conversely, some clients might feel uneasy and ask for a therapist rather than a student to help with their transfers.

Bringing clients into the decision-making process shows respect for "recipients of service" and follows the AOTA Code of Ethics Principle 3, Autonomy, Privacy and Confidentiality, which says practitioners should inform clients of the potential outcomes of service and respect their right to refuse service. By dealing with this situation in the same way for all fieldwork students, special attention is not called to Christine and the impression is not given that she cannot handle the usual student training assignments.

There must be trust and faithfulness between the practitioner and his client, and a dilemma arises when the practitioner has doubts about the skills and abilities of his student. Given the solution just discussed, the fieldwork supervisor is able to carry out his duty of providing a safe environment for client treatment, and he can feel more comfortable if clients are given the opportunity to make decisions about the safe conditions of their treatment.

Christine is merely asking for a chance. She has demonstrated that she can transfer clients safely, and the fieldwork supervisor must allow her to perform transfers, although he may justifiably monitor her during the task. If she successfully demonstrates a continued ability to transfer clients safely by the midpoint of her fieldwork experience, she should be allowed to continue without close supervision.

The academic fieldwork coordinator might have negotiated this plan or something similar with Christine and her supervisor. One of the aims of the academic coordinator is to stave off adversarial situations at fieldwork sites. Working closely with the fieldwork supervisor to construct a plan such as this one would achieve that outcome. Students could enjoy their right to a beneficial training program while learning their duty to respect clients' rights to refuse treatment, and the fieldwork supervisor could feel confident that he was maintaining his duty regarding the safety and well-being of his clients. Meanwhile, the solution is in keeping with the AOTA Code of Ethics as well as the spirit and letter of the ADA.

Study Questions

1. Define the term disability under the Americans with Disabilities Act.

2. By what criteria is it a breach of confidentiality to inform employers of an individual's disability?

3. When attending a job interview, when is an individual considered an "otherwise qualified individual" under the ADA?

4. Identify two essential and two nonessential job functions for an occupational therapist. Give your rationale.

5. Why is it both illegal and unethical to segregate the job duties of an otherwise qualified occupational therapy student or practitioner?

Gates into Practice

CASE: **Affiliating Fieldwork Student Believes She Is Infected with HIV**

with commentaries by **Mary E. Evenson, MPH, OTR, and Penny Kyler, MA, OTR, FAOTA**

Key Terms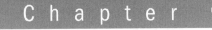

AIDS
Exposure-prone procedures
HIV

The HIV antibody test
Universal Precautions

CASE: Affiliating Fieldwork Student Believes She Is Infected with HIV

Margaret is expected to graduate summa cum laude in May. She is finishing her last six weeks of fieldwork on an oncology unit. Her daily responsibilities include assessing individuals who have some form of cancer. Margaret has been having monogamous, intimate sexual contact with a heterosexual man who recently learned he is infected with the human immunodeficiency virus **(HIV).** Her partner has regularly used condoms, but Margaret is worried that she may have been exposed to HIV. She is afraid to discuss this issue with her parents because they are devoutly religious people who are opposed to premarital sex.

Margaret is in a panic. She has no appointment and bursts into the academic fieldwork coordinator's office. The student shares her predicament with the coordinator. What should the fieldwork coordinator do? The student, having a reasonable basis for believing she is infected with HIV, is properly seeking help. What is an appropriate response to provide for both the student's health and educational needs and the welfare of clients in the clinical setting? Who should the fieldwork coordinator contact, and how should confidentiality be handled? What is the university's obligation to the oncology unit, to the clients served by Margaret, and to the student herself, who may be at risk for secondary infections if her immune status is compromised as a result of HIV? What is the student's ethical and legal responsibility to the clinical program? Margaret is expected to receive a special award at the university's graduation ceremony, and there is concern that any alteration in her fieldwork assignment may bring unwarranted media attention.

At this point, Margaret has not been tested for the HIV antibody. Pending state laws and the policies and procedures of both the healthcare facilities and the university, Margaret is uncertain if there are differences in how various aspects of confidentiality and proceeding with further steps are to be handled. The fieldwork coordinator is also concerned that the student reports having lacerated her finger while splinting a client on her previous fieldwork placement. Must this incident now be reported? By whom and to whom? In these instances, how can discriminatory actions be avoided while the clients under this student's care are reasonably and responsibly protected?

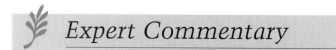

Expert Commentary

By Mary E. Evenson, MPH, OTR

The fear of contagion is linked to the fear of one's own mortality (Pizzi, 1990, p. 199).

Evolving Epidemic

The prevalence of HIV and/or acquired immune deficiency syndrome **(AIDS)** is believed to affect at least 900,000 Americans (Centers for Disease Control and Prevention [CDC], 2001a, p. 49). Furthermore, in terms of incidence, it is estimated that approximately 40,000 individuals in the United States become infected with HIV each year (CDC, 2001a, p. 7) (Box 4-1). This number has been relatively stable since 1992 but remains unacceptably high (CDC, 2001a, p. 1). It is estimated that approximately one-half of all new HIV infections are among people age 25 and younger, and most are infected sexually (CDC, 2001a, p. 18).

Overall, it is believed that the incidence and prevalence of individuals with

Box 4-1 *Summary*

HIV and/or AIDS affects at least 900,000 Americans. Approximately 40,000 individuals become infected with HIV each year.

HIV remains underreported because of the stigma and the fear of social consequences of being diagnosed with HIV/AIDS. In addition, variations in state laws affecting confidentiality and reporting procedures for monitoring cases of HIV and/or AIDS have complicated efforts aimed at an accurate epidemiological survey of HIV/AIDS. It is hoped that more accurate reporting will provide additional information about HIV-infected populations to enhance efforts to prevent HIV transmission, improve allocation of resources for treatment services, and assist in evaluating the effect of public health interventions (CDC, 1999). With advances in antiretroviral therapy and the implementation of new HIV treatment guidelines, early detection and initiation of treatment are crucial steps to allay the disease progression.

Thus the case of a fieldwork student who believes she is infected with HIV is a timely and complex predicament that raises many public health, ethical, legal, and emotional issues for occupational therapy practitioners. Public health guidelines and healthcare regulations on the prevention of HIV transmission tend to focus on the potential occupational hazards for healthcare workers (Box 4-2). Healthcare workers' procedures have been analyzed and designated at higher risk for transmission of HIV and hepatitis B virus (HBV) during exposure-prone invasive procedures such as dental work, surgery, general medical practice, obstetrics and gynecology, and cardiac and trauma services (CDC, 1991). The rights of healthcare workers, their confidentiality, and their "right to know" the HIV status of the patient versus the patient's right to confidentiality continues to be debated (Blatchford et al., 2000) (Box 4-3). How can everyone's rights and confidentiality be protected?

Do clients have a need and a right to know whether an occupational therapy practitioner or occupational therapy student is HIV positive, even if the intervention, as in most occupational therapy practice, does not involve performing exposure-prone invasive procedures and the risk of exchanging blood? As health professionals, occupational therapy practitioners must base reactions to this question on contemporary scientific evidence together with a thoughtful analysis of the interrelationships between the risks involved and the rights of individuals. Moreover, adherence to the highest standards of professional conduct and behavior is essential. Although these standards are necessary, they are insufficient by themselves to answer complex ethical and legal questions. What does scientific information tell us about HIV transmission from healthcare worker to client, and what are the professional standards in this case?

Box 4-2 *Summary*

In the workplace, public health guidelines and healthcare regulations on prevention of HIV transmission tend to focus on the potential hazards for healthcare workers.

Box 4-3 *Ethical Dilemma*

The rights of healthcare workers, their confidentiality, and their right to know the HIV status of their clients versus the client's right to confidentiality continues to be debated.

How can the rights of the possibly HIV-positive student be balanced with the legitimate concerns of the client and fieldwork center?

Margaret's situation directs concerns to the issues of confidentiality, testing for HIV, discrimination, client protection, the professional responsibility of the occupational therapy student and the academic fieldwork coordinator, the legal and ethical responsibilities of the university and healthcare settings, and HIV and AIDS education. Moreover, although these issues parallel issues concerning a professional with HIV infection, student status presents unique problems. The professional has already completed certification requirements and will have access to a variety of career opportunities if clinical practice is not an option. The occupational therapy student must complete fieldwork experiences to meet the eligibility requirements for the national certification examination and future entry into practice.

Margaret's case presents many complex issues. This chapter addresses these issues within the context of a rapidly changing social, cultural, and scientific environment where knowledge, attitudes, research, and technology are still emerging. As advances occur, the appropriateness of particular ethical, legal, and professional views may vary.

The Role of the Academic Fieldwork Coordinator

The response to Margaret is influenced by the personal and professional values of all the people involved. HIV challenges all healthcare practitioners because it forces us to examine our personal values concerning sexuality and mortality. The academic fieldwork coordinator may want to pause to note the feelings that Margaret's situation raises for him or her. We need to examine our biases and fears and make them explicit, at least in our own minds, to minimize a potentially biased response.

The academic fieldwork coordinator has professional, ethical, and legal obligations to the student, the fieldwork education setting, and the university. An important component of the academic fieldwork coordinator's role is to teach and model professional behavior, judgment, and decision making; to educate the student about HIV and AIDS; and to adhere to the responsibilities outlined in the memorandum of agreement (Box 4-4).

In most situations, occupational therapy academic programs sign a memorandum of agreement with each fieldwork education institution. These agreements outline the responsibilities of both parties and include guidelines for students' health status with the students' informed and written consent. The academic program often agrees to send the fieldwork education institution a copy of students' health sta-

Box 4-4 *Summary*

The academic fieldwork coordinator has professional, ethical, and legal obligations to the student, the fieldwork setting, and the university. An important component of the academic fieldwork coordinator's role is to teach and model professional behavior, judgment, and decision making, and to educate the student about the HIV and AIDS.

tus reports. These confidential reports document the results of students' complete physical examinations and immunizations for polio, rubella, measles, mumps, and hepatitis B. Most memoranda of agreement include a clause that states that students may be withdrawn from the fieldwork program if their health status is a detriment to the clients or to their successful completion of the fieldwork program. The memoranda of agreement need to be carefully reviewed before making any determination regarding Margaret's status because legal terms may vary from state to state and among institutions.

The academic program is also responsible for notifying each student that he or she is responsible for following the administrative policies, standards, regulations, and practice of the fieldwork education institution. In addition, students must conform to standards and practices outlined by the academic program and university while completing the fieldwork component of their professional education. This includes conforming to the American Occupational Therapy Association (AOTA) Code of Ethics (AOTA, 2000a). Finally, the agreements require all parties to abide by policies of nondiscrimination determined by each respective institution.

Confidentiality

The most immediate concern is attending to the panic that Margaret has expressed. She will need guidance in determining a responsible course of action that embraces the professional ethics of occupational therapy and adheres to the university standards. Furthermore, she will need reassurance that maintaining her confidentiality is one of the highest priorities of the university and the academic fieldwork coordinator. Potential adverse social and professional consequences are attached to being publicly identified as being HIV positive, which makes respect for confidentiality so important (Box 4-5). As a result, the CDC now requires that recipients of federal funding for HIV/AIDS surveillance establish policies in accordance with the recommended minimum security standards to protect confidentiality. These standards state that HIV/AIDS surveillance data must not include names of individuals or other identifying information and that data must be located in a physically secured area using coded passwords and computer encryption to protect data records (CDC, 1999) (Box 4-6). The HIV/AIDS Bureau of the Health Resources and Services Administration,

Box 4-5 *Ethical Dilemma*

Potential adverse social and professional consequences are attached to being publicly identified as being HIV positive, which makes confidentiality extremely important.

Box 4-6 *By the Law*

Margaret's right to privacy and confidentiality is protected by:

▶ The Centers for Disease Control and Prevention
▶ The HIV/AIDS Bureau of the Health Resources and Services Administration
▶ The AOTA Code of Ethics
▶ The Family Educational Rights and Privacy Act

which funds states to develop and provide services for the uninsured and underinsured, also mandates grantees to protect the confidentiality of those they serve (Box 4-6).

Professionally, Margaret's privacy must be protected. The AOTA Code of Ethics, Principle 7A (AOTA, 2000a) states that: "Occupational therapy personnel shall preserve, respect, and safeguard confidential information about colleagues and staff, unless otherwise mandated by national, state, or local laws" (p. 615). However, the potential risks to the third parties must also be evaluated (Box 4-6).

The Family Educational Rights and Privacy Act (1974), known as FERPA or the Buckley Amendment, also protects Margaret's right to privacy pertaining to her matriculation within an educational institution (Box 4-6). This amendment is designed to guarantee students access to their own personal education records while preventing unauthorized persons from accessing these records without the student's consent. The academic fieldwork coordinator cannot release private information about a student unless the student gives the coordinator written consent to do so. Health records or health information is considered private information. Although FERPA protects access to Margaret's educational record, there is no need to document Margaret's situation at this time because there is no evidence that could affect her education. The coordinator needs to explore with Margaret with whom she has shared this information and explain that it is private information and that she has the right to keep it private.

Although Margaret's right to privacy is a top priority, these rights are not absolute. There are other considerations. Healthcare workers have a moral obligation not to harm their clients. What level of risk to the client is involved must be determined. Even if the risk of harm to the client is miniscule, to what degree does the risk warrant violating Margaret's moral right to keep her HIV status confidential? Her HIV status is unknown. Therefore, there is no indication to share her potential HIV status at this time.

Initial Determination: Emotional Stability

Before the potential risk involved in transmitting the virus to clients is assessed, the following questions might be posed: Why is Margaret sharing this information? How will this potential threat to her own health affect her ability to provide health care for others, especially her current clients who are confronting their own mortality? Given that this situation raises numerous highly charged emotional issues for Margaret, such as her own mortality, her relationship with her boyfriend and her family, and her sexuality, it needs to be determined whether she is emotionally prepared to continue the fieldwork experience. This question is further complicated by the vulnerability of the oncology clinical population with whom Margaret is currently working. Common forms of cancer such as breast cancer and cervical or ovarian cancer all raise issues regarding sexuality for the clients.

Will Margaret be able to provide the quality of care these clients clearly deserve? How will Margaret integrate and cope with this information in her life? Perhaps Margaret should even be temporarily suspended from fieldwork. Answers to some of these questions may require the expertise of trained mental health professionals. Given that issues of confidentiality have already been reviewed with Margaret, the coordinator may contract with Margaret to meet with staff from the university counseling center to determine her emotional readiness to continue the fieldwork experience. Because her HIV status is unknown at this time, any determination related to continuing the fieldwork placement would be based on the recommendations from the counseling center regarding her emotional stability and potential to direct her attention to providing quality care for her clients.

Testing for HIV

Of primary concern is the goal of increasing the percentage of those already infected in the United States to know they are infected through voluntary counseling and testing, especially in regard to early detection, as outlined in the *HIV Prevention Strategic Plan through 2005* (CDC, 2001a). This plan states:

> HIV counseling should not be a barrier to HIV testing, and testing should not be a barrier to counseling. Counseling and testing strategies for those who deny their risk, those who recognize their risk but have not been tested and those who underestimate or are unaware of their risk will all be different. (p. 34)

Reasons for seeking HIV testing are often associated with services offered for pregnant women, clients at sexually transmitted disease clinics, those donating blood, military service screening, and those persons who present with symptoms of HIV-related illness (CDC, 1999).

Margaret will need information about the availability of options for confidential and anonymous HIV/AIDS testing programs and other resources in the area. It is not the role of the university counseling staff or the academic fieldwork coordinator to decide whether Margaret should be tested. Rather, they are responsible for explaining testing procedures and reminding her of any university or fieldwork institution guidelines that outline students' responsibilities. Fear of discrimination may create a reluctance to be tested. Loss of a future career, Margaret's relationship with her parents, and other emotionally charged issues may provide a disincentive to seeking testing. Because HIV/AIDS testing has the potential to cause emotional, social, and legal problems, counseling is an integral component of the testing procedure in many healthcare centers (Box 4-7).

Box 4-7 **Summary**

Because HIV/AIDS testing has the potential to cause emotional, social, and legal problems, counseling should be an integral component of the testing procedure.

The initial counseling session should:

► Help [Margaret] understand what the test can and can't tell her.

► Explain issues of confidentiality and the procedure used to guarantee privacy.

► Help assess the risk of exposure to the AIDS virus by offering information about high-risk sexual and drug-taking behavior.

► Help [Margaret] make a plan to deal with either positive or negative test results.

► Give [Margaret] names and phone numbers of people she can contact if she has questions or concerns while waiting for test results. (Hopp & Rogers, 1989, p. 292)

► Further discussion during a counseling session should:

► Explain treatment options if test results are positive.

► Ensure an understanding of safe-sex practices until test results are known.

► Coach [Margaret] in communication with her partner.

► Explore postexposure testing and treatment options and resources.

(Y. Glendon, personal communication, October 3, 2001)

In regard to longer-term concerns, Margaret will need information or access to counseling about the implications of positive or negative testing for her career and future health, personal issues with her boyfriend and family, and other psychosocial concerns. Anonymous testing centers are available in many locations and by mail. The test can be taken without providing a name, address, telephone number, social security number, or other information that might be used to trace test results in the future. Anonymous testing guarantees that no one else can know the test results without the person's permission. Accordingly, a code number is assigned to each client to identify the blood sample. In fact, some states offer free anonymous testing and counseling. Centers offering these free services are referred to as alternative test sites. Local health departments have a listing of the alternative test sites in their area (Hopp & Rogers, 1989). In addition, the CDC has a national hotline for AIDS information (1-800-342-AIDS).

If Margaret proceeds with HIV testing, there are some important facts for her to keep in mind during the 6-month interim following her initial test. The HIV antibody test does not screen blood for the AIDS virus. The test screens for the antibodies associated with AIDS, that of HIV. A positive test result identifies whether an individual has been exposed to the virus associated with AIDS but cannot identify whether that person has a virus in his or her system (Box 4-8). Therefore, the test will not indicate when or if the person might become ill. Conversely, a negative test result means no HIV antibodies have been found in the blood. These antibodies are often not detectable for up to six months after exposure to the virus, so it is possible to be infected by the virus yet have no sign of antibodies in the blood. Consequently, a negative test

Box 4-8 *Summary*

The HIV antibody test screens for antibodies associated with HIV. It does not screen for the AIDS virus. A positive test indicates only that an individual has been exposed to HIV but will not indicate if the virus is currently in the individual's system.

result does *not* mean that a person can't be infected in the future. Therefore, test results cannot be relied on to guide behavior. Negative test results may create only an illusion of security because it may take up to six months for the body to undergo seroconversion (development of evidence of antibody response to a disease). Whether the test is positive or negative, behavior and decision making should be the same. **Universal Precautions** should be used at all times because it is difficult to know a true HIV antibody status (Hopp & Rogers, 1989; Martelli, Peltz, & Messina, 1987).

Whatever the outcome of the HIV testing, Margaret may also need post-test counseling. A clear understanding of the test results will facilitate Margaret's ability to cope with her situation. This counseling may be provided through the alternative test site or the university counseling center. Most important, Margaret should be connected to the available resources. She may also need resources or referral sources for her boyfriend. It is not the academic fieldwork coordinator's role to find services for the boyfriend, but this issue may be important for Margaret. Finally, it is important to note that even if Margaret does pursue testing, it is ultimately her choice to share the test results.

Guideline Review

To respond to this situation, keeping in mind current knowledge concerning HIV transmission and professional standards, the academic fieldwork coordinator should review existing professional, university, federal, and local guidelines, which are discussed as follows.

Universal Precautions

The nature of the clinical activity and the student's understanding and adherence to the Universal Precautions for Prevention of Transmission of HIV, HBV, and Other Bloodborne Pathogens in Health Care Settings, developed by the CDC in 1988, are essential factors to consider in making any determination regarding Margaret's situation (Box 4-9). The best methods of preventing the spread of HIV to patients are set forth in these guidelines. The CDC (1991) concludes:

Box 4-9 *Summary*

It is essential that all healthcare workers adhere to the Universal Precautions for Prevention and Transmission of HIV, HBV, and Other Bloodborne Pathogens in Health Care Settings, developed by the CDC in 1988.

Investigations of HIV and HBV (Hepatitis B) transmission from health care workers to patients indicates that, when healthcare workers adhere to recommended infection-control procedures, the risk of transmitting HBV from an infected health care worker to a patient is small, and the risk of transmitting HIV is likely to be even smaller. (p. 4)

Adherence to Universal Precautions, including appropriate use of handwashing, protective barriers, and care in the use and disposal of needles and other sharp instruments, can greatly reduce the risk of healthcare worker injury and the risk of transmission of not just HIV but all bloodborne pathogens. HBV is much more easily transmitted than AIDS and has been recognized for a longer time. Thus, if all healthcare professionals strictly adhere to these guidelines for every patient, this will provide maximal protection and minimal discrimination for all. The CDC asserts that proper application of the principles of Universal Precautions will assist in minimizing the risk of transmission of HIV or HBV from patient to healthcare worker, from healthcare worker to patient, and from patient to patient (CDC, 1991).

Universal Precautions are designed and intended to be practiced when delivering care to *all* individuals, not only for clients with AIDS or other infectious conditions. Given the importance of adhering to Universal Precautions in healthcare settings, all occupational therapy programs should routinely educate their students in proper infection control procedures. Ideally, all healthcare workers who might be at risk for exposure to blood in a work setting should receive HBV vaccinations, preferably during professional training, before any occupational exposures could occur. Therefore, assume that Margaret has been educated in the use of Universal Precautions, has received an HBV vaccination, and follows these Universal Precaution guidelines in her fieldwork placements.

Retrospective Studies: Magnitude of the Risk

With the onset of HIV and AIDS in the United States in the 1980s, the fear and concern of HIV transmission from healthcare worker to client received widespread attention in the popular media. As a result, the CDC instituted epidemiologic survey programs in an effort to research and track HIV transmissions to identify potential patterns of risk in relation to specific populations as well as specific healthcare practices. As professionals, a review of current knowledge regarding the risks must be factored into a response to Margaret.

Since June 2002, approximately 23,500 reported cases of adults with AIDS have been employed in health care in the United States. These cases represent 5.1 percent of the AIDS cases reported to the CDC for whom occupational information was known. Overall, 73 percent of the healthcare workers with AIDS, including 1,374 physicians, 87 surgeons, 3,791 nurses, 378 dental workers, and 315 paramedics, are reported to have died (CDC, 2002b).

Occupational exposures have resulted in 57 documented cases of HIV seroconversion among healthcare workers in the United States as of June 2001. Of these individuals, 26 have developed AIDS. The individuals who seroconverted include 19 laboratory workers, 24 nurses, 6 physicians, 2 surgical technicians, 1 dialysis technician, 1 respiratory technician, 1 health aide, 1 embalmer technician, and 2 housekeeper/ maintenance workers. The CDC has developed recommendations for preventing transmission of HIV and HBV to patients and states that "Infected health care workers who adhere to Universal Precautions and who do not perform invasive procedures pose no risk for transmitting HIV or HBV to patients" (CDC, 1991). Furthermore, it is advised that "health care workers who have exudative lesions or weeping dermatitis should refrain from all direct patient care and from handling patient-care equipment and devices used in performing invasive procedures until the condition resolves" (CDC, 1991).

The CDC (1991) has compiled studies of HIV infections among healthcare workers who performed invasive exposure-prone procedures. One investigation reveals that a dentist with AIDS likely transmitted HIV to approximately 5 of 850 patients evaluated through 1991. In two other studies, 75 patients cared for by a general surgeon with AIDS and 62 patients cared for by a surgical resident with AIDS all tested negative. A fourth study of a dental student with HIV showed negative tests for HIV infection among all 143 patients who had been treated. There is limited ability to generalize this information because of the small number of participants in these studies as well as the differences in procedures associated with particular medical practices.

These studies imply minimal need to restrict the work of healthcare workers infected with HIV, especially when appropriate infection control procedures are followed (Weiss, 1992). These data are important to consider when evaluating Margaret's situation. The significance of the current understanding is that it is difficult to actually contract HIV from a healthcare worker who does not perform invasive procedures.

Professional Guidelines

The preventive strategies recommended by the CDC encourage healthcare workers to assume that blood and other body fluids from all patients are potentially infectious. Therefore, infection control precautions should be followed at all times. These precautions include the following:

- ▶ The routine use of barriers (such as gloves and/or goggles) when anticipating contact with blood or body fluids
- ▶ Washing hands and other skin surfaces immediately after contact with blood or body fluids
- ▶ Careful handling and disposing of sharp instruments during and after use

(CDC, 2002a)

Although education and prevention are felt to be most important in reducing the risk of occupational exposures, having a plan in place for postexposure management of healthcare personnel is essential. Recommendations for Post Exposure Prophylaxis (PEP) have been published (CDC, June 19, 2001b), and occupational exposures should be considered urgent medical concerns. In most cases of HIV exposure that warrant PEP, a basic two-drug regimen is recommended for four weeks. In the instance of an increased risk, a three-drug regimen may be recommended. Healthcare workers should continue to practice Universal Precautions with extra vigilance following an exposure as well as practicing PEP and safe-sex practices with a partner until 6-month postexposure testing proves negative.

The AOTA does not have specific guidelines for HIV-positive practitioners because occupational therapy practitioners are not typically involved in invasive or exposure-prone procedures. In a position paper on HIV, however, the AOTA does recommend that "occupational therapy practitioners adhere to appropriate infection control procedures as defined by their facility and by local, state, and federal regulations" (AOTA, 1989a, p. 1) (Box 4-10). Although the reference is to HIV-infected clients, they point out that when such precautions are implemented, persons with HIV do not present a health risk to others. Other professionals who are regularly involved in invasive procedures have given these dilemmas serious consideration. For example, the American Dental Association policy requires determining actions involving HIV-infected dental healthcare workers on a case-by-case basis to avoid endangering patients or members of the dental staff (American Dental Association, 1991). The U.S. Public Health Service, the American Hospital Association, state hospital associations, and state public health departments similarly advocate individual assessments to determine patient care duties of HIV-infected healthcare workers (Gostin, 1989).

Box 4-10 **By the Law**

AOTA recommends that occupational therapy practitioners adhere to appropriate infection control policies as defined by their facility and by local, state, and federal regulators.

Local Guidelines

It is believed that government regulation of healthcare professionals is necessary "to protect the public from incompetent and unethical practitioners" (Sultz & Young, 2001, p. 171). The U.S. Senate and House of Representatives passed legislation that allows each state to adopt different rules for healthcare workers (Hilts, 1991) Thus, it would be important to understand a particular state's regulations. Given variations among state laws, it is most important to evaluate the nature of the clinical activity and the miniscule risk that Margaret could pose to her clients' health.

University and Federal Guidelines

In Margaret's situation, if her university has an established policy on AIDS, the academic fieldwork coordinator should follow those guidelines. Faculty and students are responsible for being familiar with and following the university policy and guidelines, as well as any policy of the affiliated fieldwork institutions where they are responsible for providing client care services. The rights and responsibilities of the HIV-positive student are usually outlined in such policies. Voluntary disclosure on a confidential basis is written into these policies, because any individual who is at risk for AIDS or who knows that he or she is HIV positive has a moral obligation to take all possible steps to prevent harm to others (Bayer, Levine, & Wolf, 1986).

As previously recommended, academic programs should require all students to attend an infectious disease informational session in which guidelines are presented. Thus, if Margaret has attended such training, she will be familiar with the university policies. Then if she does test positive for HIV, she should be encouraged to voluntarily disclose her status as outlined in the university guidelines.

University polices usually identify a designated official or expert review panel who determine on a case-by-case basis the risks posed by the HIV-infected student. In Margaret's case, the academic fieldwork coordinator should recommend that Margaret notify the panel at her university. If Margaret was unable to notify the panel herself, the academic fieldwork coordinator should obtain written consent to present Margaret's case for her. Such a panel follows the recommendations set forth in the CDC guidelines, which state that infected healthcare workers should appear before a special review panel, to determine under what circumstances they would be able to continue practice.

The CDC guidelines (1991) state that the panel should be composed of experts who represent a balanced perspective and who counsel the infected healthcare worker who performs exposure-prone procedures. Specifically, it is suggested that:

> Experts might include all of the following: a) the health care worker's personal physician(s), b) an infectious disease specialist with expertise in the epidemiology of HIV and HBV transmission, c) a health professional with expertise in the procedures performed by the health care worker, and d) state or local public health official(s) . . . [and] a member of the infection-control committee, preferably a hospital epidemiologist.
>
> (CDC, 1991)

These guidelines are helpful for healthcare institutions, although translation to an academic institution makes implementation challenging. Suggested panel participants within the university might include the academic fieldwork coordinator, department chairperson and/or dean, university health services staff, risk management staff, and legal counsel. Because there is no definitive statement from the CDC regarding the panel's power to summon people or make binding decisions, the whole procedure is "voluntary in the sense that the infected health care worker has the choice of revealing his or her condition to such a panel" (O'Rourke & de Blois, 1991, p.41). Furthermore, consulting such a panel raises concerns regarding confidentiality. As more people become aware of the situation, it becomes more difficult to ensure confidentiality. Respecting a person's right to privacy requires that those privileged to such information maintain its confidentiality. This panel should be bound by strict confidentiality and make every effort to guard Margaret's privacy.

Central to this panel would be the determination of what constitutes an "invasive" or **"exposure-prone procedure."** The CDC guidelines for preventing transmission of HIV to patients state that those practitioners who test positive for HIV should refrain from invasive procedures, including certain oral, cardiothoracic, colorectal, and obstetric/gynecologic procedures, as well as general and orthopedic surgeries, and trauma services. The guidelines generally state that "exposure prone procedures involve digital palpation of a needle tip in a body cavity or the simultaneous presence of the health care worker's fingers and a needle or other sharp instruments or objects in a poorly visualized or highly confined anatomical site" (CDC, 1991). Overall, medical, surgical, and dental facilities should identify which procedures performed are to be considered exposure-prone. These general definitions force practitioners to address each healthcare worker who is infected with HIV on a case-by-case basis.

The CDC (1991) guidelines explicitly state, however, that there is no basis for restricting the practice of HIV-infected healthcare workers in performing noninvasive procedures or procedures that are not exposure-prone. If Margaret tests positive for HIV and then chooses to disclose her status to a university panel, they may want to review the CDC guidelines with Margaret and identify the types of interventions she is using with clients in her present fieldwork placement. Of primary concern would be whether Margaret is involved in any activity that would be considered invasive or exposure-prone.

Because most standards for decisions about disclosure raise the question of degree of risk or level of invasiveness, the interventions used in Margaret's setting must be carefully examined. A comprehensive text of occupational therapy practice (Neistadt & Crepeau, 1998) reviews the interventions that occupational therapy practitioners use in a hospital setting with clients who have been diagnosed with cancer immediately following surgery, or during chemotherapy or radiation treatment. The general purpose of an occupational therapy referral may often be to evaluate and provide interventions to improve basic self-care and mobility abilities. "Swallowing may also be an issue if the person develops dysphagia from neurological damage, surgical resection involving the oral or oral pharyngeal cavity, or fungal infections of the oral pharyngeal cavity" (Pizzi & Burkhardt, 1998, p. 712).

Once the client with cancer has completed initial medical procedures and treatment regimens, referral for additional occupational therapy services may address joint mobility limitations, lymphedema, loss or impairment of upper extremity and hand function, scar management, splinting, and positioning, fabrication of cosmetic or assistive devices, alterations in body image, depression, an adjustment disorder, or somatosensory pain syndromes. With advancing late stages of disease, the focus of intervention becomes that of comfort or palliative care. Here, the role of the practitioner is to support clients in meeting their emotional needs while striving to maintain some degree of mastery over the environment.

These interventions do not typically involve invasive or exposure-prone procedures, with the exception of interventions for dysphagia and scar management if the wound is not fully healed. As a result, the panel will need to rely on accurate reporting from the fieldwork site, Margaret, and the academic fieldwork coordinator to fully understand the expectation of Margaret's specific client care duties. If it is determined that Margaret is involved in invasive or exposure-prone procedures, such as dysphagia evaluation and interventions, the panel must determine if her fieldwork practices should be modified or restricted to prevent the risk of infection transmission. If, however, it is determined that Margaret is not involved in invasive or exposure-prone procedures, the panel must ask if she is any more likely to sustain needlestick and sharp injuries than are experienced professionals.

An additional question for the panel to explore is whether Margaret has an increased potential for causing invasive injuries to clients accidentally. It is unlikely that Margaret would cause invasive injuries accidentally because occupational therapy practitioners do not routinely use sharp instruments in their interventions. Finally, and perhaps most important, the panel should determine Margaret's ability to follow proper infection control standards.

In the unlikely event that it was determined that Margaret was involved in invasive or exposure-prone procedures and posed significant risk of transmitting HIV infection to her clients, she would be bound by the professional standard not to harm the clients she treats. Principle 2 of the AOTA Code of Ethics (AOTA, 2000a, p. 614) states that: "Occupational therapy personnel shall take reasonable precautions to avoid imposing or inflicting harm upon the recipient of services or to his or her property." Gostin (1989), in a well-thought-out paper on HIV infection and invasive procedures, argues that students may be acting negligently if they continue to practice when they know, or reasonably should know, that their physical condition may pose a risk for the client.

Thus, if after a thorough process of review, the academic program's panel determines that Margaret does pose a significant risk of transmission to clients, the school would have four options:

1. The academic program could recommend that the university dismiss Margaret and make HIV testing available at no charge to her present and former clients. Although this option would satisfy the professional responsibility to protect the well-being of a third party, it might violate Margaret's right to privacy

because that action would increase the possibility that her identity would be revealed. This approach also violates the value of a basic moral principle of respect for autonomy or self-determination because Margaret would no longer be free to pursue her occupational therapy education.

2.   A second option would allow Margaret to continue her field-work placement while protecting her confidentiality. Although this option protects Margaret's right to privacy, there is a risk of endangering her clients.

3.   A similar approach to the second option is to recommend continuing the fieldwork while Margaret modifies her client interventions. This alternative could help minimize potential risks to Margaret's clients by forbidding her to perform procedures that might risk skin lacerations or mucous transmissions during interventions for dysphagia and scar management.

4.   A fourth option would involve removing Margaret from direct client care activities. If the school were to take such an action, they would be fulfilling their obligation to protect the safety of clients. Because Margaret has a right to privacy, the university would need to be more prudent in its efforts to maintain Margaret's confidentiality. The right to decide to whom information may be disclosed belongs to Margaret, not university employees. Ideally, university staff would actively involve Margaret in the decision-making process or at the very least discuss the panel's recommendation with her. Can Margaret be suspended from her fieldwork placement pending a hearing? According to Weinstein and Keyes (1991), such actions would likely meet judicial approval if the school's panel can make a legitimate argument that the suspension was based on concerns for client safety.

If it were determined that a potential risk of transmitting the HIV infection to clients existed, the hospital, occupational therapy fieldwork supervisor, and former clients would have to be notified. It would be important for the review panel to determine exactly who needs to know this information and to make every effort to ensure that those without a need to know would not be informed of Margaret's identity. According to the American Bar Association, it would be important to obtain written informed consent from Margaret to disclose this information (Rennert, 1991). The written consent should include (1) the individuals or agency to receive the information, (2) the time period during which the consent is effective, (3) Margaret's right to revoke consent, (4) precisely what information the university is authorized to disclose, and (5) the purpose of the disclosure.

Notification could be sent via certified letters with restricted delivery informing the hospital, occupational therapy fieldwork supervisor, and former clients that one of their former occupational therapy students was HIV positive. The clients should be told that the likelihood of possible transmission was extremely low and that testing for the presence of the HIV antibody is recommended. The academic program should identify resources for testing and make the appropriate arrangements (Comer et al., 1991).

If Margaret were removed from clinical activities, both the Americans with Disabilities Act (ADA, 1990) and Section 504 of the Rehabilitation Act of 1973 raise concerns related to reasonable accommodation for Margaret. These pieces of legislation extend federal civil rights protections to those who have or are perceived to have disabilities, including HIV infection. They provide qualified students who have documented disabilities access to the same quality of education and the same expectations for performance available to other students. It is expected that reasonable accommodations (i.e., efforts to make adjustments for impairments) will be made by all programs receiving federal monies.

Koelbl (1992), in his discussion of HIV-positive dental students, points out that from a legal standpoint an HIV-infected dental student would be considered a handicapped individual. Given this perspective, questions arise regarding whether Margaret would be considered a handicapped individual who was otherwise qualified to become an occupational therapist and, if so, what accommodations are required by the academic program? For dental students, the issues are somewhat clearer because most dental procedures are invasive.

> If there is a significant risk of transmission of HIV from student to patients, then the student is probably not otherwise qualified to perform invasive procedures. This position is supported by the ADA policy, which states that HIV-infected dentists should refrain from performing invasive procedures.
>
> (Koelbl, 1992, p. 17)

In the case of healthcare workers whose practices have been modified because of HIV or HBV infection status, it is highly recommended that workers be provided opportunities to continue appropriate client care activities whenever possible. Supportive resources such as job retraining and/or career counseling should be made available to enable the individual's continued use of talents, skills, and knowledge (CDC, 1991). In the instance of healthcare workers with HBV, periodic reevaluation of hepatitis B status changes are indicated because of the possible resolution of infection in response to treatment.

In occupational therapy, it is not clear that practitioners are involved in invasive or exposure-prone procedures, and there may be alternatives in a clinical setting, such as providing noninvasive procedures to a low-risk population. Therefore, it is unclear whether Margaret would be handicapped or otherwise qualified if she were removed from the oncology unit fieldwork placement.

Laws aside, ethical standards related to what practitioners ought to do might help the university panel make a decision regarding accommodations for Margaret. Margaret probably could be accommodated by identifying alternative roles within the profession of occupational therapy. Flexibility and adaptation are central tenets of the profession, and these values should be applied to Margaret as well as to the clients for whom practitioners provide services.

Former Client Contact

Complicating the case even further, Margaret reports having lacerated her finger while splinting a client on her previous fieldwork placement. Healthcare workers who cut or puncture themselves do not necessarily expose the client to their blood. Friedland and Klein (1987) report that a small inoculum of contaminated blood is unlikely to transmit HIV. There is no need to draw undue attention to the potential risk until it is determined that Margaret has received positive HIV test results. Even if there is a miniscule risk that Margaret infected her former client, the university's expert review panel would have to consider this incident as well. If she does test positive for HIV, it would be important to find out more details about the incident. Were appropriate precautions followed? How severe was the laceration? Was the blood contained? What was the client's diagnosis, and did the client have any open wounds? Was Margaret's fieldwork supervisor present during this potential exposure? If not, did Margaret inform her fieldwork supervisor? Was an incident report completed and filed with the fieldwork facility's risk management department? These are just a few of the many questions that need exploration.

The review panel also has some options. One option would be to assume that there is no chance that Margaret exposed her former client to blood. Therefore, no action would be necessary. If it was determined that Margaret possibly transmitted the HIV infection to her former clients, they and appropriate hospital personnel would have to be notified. It is recommended that the university follows the same procedure already described (i.e., certified letters with restricted delivery).

Graduation Ceremony

Margaret is expected to receive a special award at the university's graduation ceremony. In the unlikely event of her removal from her fieldwork placement and the subsequent delay in her completing the program, university officials may be concerned that removing Margaret from her fieldwork placement may bring unwarranted media attention. It may be important to determine whether the special award is linked to successful completion of the program requirements—graduation. If so, university officials will have to determine an appropriate course of action. They, too, are bound by issues of confidentiality. If any media attention arises from this situation, the university's public relations department would also have to recognize issues of confidentiality and may counsel Margaret in her response to the media. The special review panel must maintain its commitment to protect Margaret's confidentiality.

Federal and state laws imply that the university would be subject to civil and criminal liability for breaches of confidentiality of HIV-related information (Rennert, 1991). The university should do everything possible to avoid disclosing the information about Margaret's situation to the public. In addition, the review panel has a responsibility to educate concerned university officials. The panel could use this opportunity to educate others because education is a powerful means to alleviate fears and dispel myths.

Summary

Because knowledge about the risk of HIV transmission is still emerging, the ideas presented in this chapter are not absolute. Occupational therapy practitioners must update their knowledge base and evaluate future situations based on current knowledge. Furthermore, proper infection control practices must be used at all times. In fact, the Occupational Safety and Health Administration (OSHA) recommends that education courses on infection control become a condition of relicensure and a requirement for professional certification (Miike et al., 1991). Regulatory agencies such as the Joint Commission for the Accreditation of Health Care Organizations and State Departments of Health have established policies that mandate ongoing education on bloodborne pathogens to ensure safety for all. These training standards are established to ensure quality care that "increases the likelihood of desired patient outcomes and reduces the likelihood of undesired outcomes given the current state of medical knowledge" (Sultz & Young, 2001, p. 102).

Occupational therapy educators have a responsibility to educate students in infection control procedures early in the students' educational experience and before all fieldwork. In addition, occupational therapy curricula should provide current information about HIV and AIDS and other infectious diseases, such as hepatitis B, to their students and faculty on a routine basis. Such education should address attitudes as well as provide knowledge in disease prevention. The *HIV Prevention Strategic Plan through 2005* (CDC, 2001a) outlines strategies to reduce the number of workers who are occupationally exposed to and infected with HIV as an objective under the overarching goal to "decrease by at least 50% the number of persons in the United States at high risk for acquiring or transmitting HIV by delivering targeted, sustained and evidence-based HIV prevention interventions" (p. 26). Strategies to prevent the transmission of HIV are recommended as follows:

1. Encourage the availability and use of effective engineering controls (e.g., engineered sharps injury prevention devices) and personal protective equipment (e.g., gloves) by healthcare workers.

2. Advocate for interventions in healthcare facilities (e.g., engineering controls, personal protective equipment, work practices, work

organization and health communication strategies) that are effective in reducing exposure to blood and body fluids among healthcare workers.

3. Implement surveillance systems to track the distribution and determinants of bloodborne exposures (including the surveillance of effective interventions) and their trends over time among healthcare and other exposed workers in all settings.

4. Encourage the use of work practices that reduce exposures to blood and body fluids by workers and the modification of work organization factors (e.g., staffing and management commitment to safety) that impact exposures to blood in healthcare facilities.

5. Encourage the use of health communication strategies that convey effective techniques for reducing exposure to blood and body fluids to workers.

6. Work with employers and insurers to provide information about postexposure prophylaxis and the importance of seeking appropriate and timely post-exposure counseling and testing, as well as needed treatment to workers (including emergency response workers) who are exposed to blood and body fluids.

(CDC, 2001a, p. 32)

These goals provide a comprehensive model for occupational therapy educators to follow. Education together with thoughtful analysis will help practitioners achieve the delicate balance between the emotional issues raised by the threat of HIV and current scientific information that supports precautions and practices to prevent transmission and minimize risks.

Margaret's predicament highlights the tension involved in protecting clients from possible HIV transmission and protecting Margaret's confidentiality and potential discrimination. This chapter's emphasis on confidentiality for Margaret may compete with public concerns and fears related to the possibility of healthcare workers transmitting HIV infection to clients. Although these fears are not necessarily rational or justified, they are real and must be acknowledged in an open and caring manner. The apprehension surrounding HIV infection should not be dismissed. The sensitive handling of these fears and balancing the conflicting values, ethics, and legal perspectives will remain a challenge to all practitioners in the decades ahead. The questions raised in this chapter will be debated for years to come.

Acknowledgements

The author wishes to express her appreciation to Ellen S. Cohn, ScD, EdM, OTR, FAOTA, who was the first edition author of this chapter, and her collaborator, Linette Liebling, MSPH, Boston AIDS Action Committee Board of Directors, for providing an understanding of the complex issues related to AIDS in today's society. Thanks also to Laurie Sabol, MLS, Tisch Library, Tufts University, who served as a guide through the government Websites and documents.

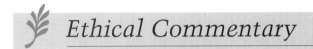

Ethical Commentary

By Penny Kyler, MA, OTR, FAOTA

The HIV/AIDS Bureau of the Health Resources and Services Administration (2002) sets out guidelines for confidentiality that state:

> Confidentiality is a major cornerstone of the therapeutic relationship. It carries special meaning for HIV-infected individuals who have experienced discrimination in the workplace and other settings, stigmatization, and occasional abandonment by friends or family. HIV-positive women may be particularly vulnerable to these effects because of lower economic status, cultural traditions and general societal beliefs about the role of women, minority status, and child care or other caretaking responsibilities. Information about a patient's HIV status or details about her medical condition should be kept strictly confidential by providers and shared only with the express permission of the woman herself. At the same time she should be encouraged and assisted in disclosing her status to others who need to know, i.e. sexual partners and health care providers.
>
> (Accessed August 13, 2002, www.hab.hrsa.gov:80/ publications/hrsawomen/chapter2/chapter2.htm)

HIV/AIDS is still a major killer. A new generation of individuals within the United States is becoming infected, as are many underserved populations in parts of Africa, Asia, and Europe. The facts of Margaret's case need clarifying to ferret out the dilemma. Margaret has not been tested for HIV; however, her concerns have led her to discuss the matter with her academic fieldwork coordinator. Following the usual format by asking the established questions, the reader should be able to sort out the facts and get to the root of the dilemma.

Who Are the Players?

The players are Margaret—a student, her sex partner, the academic fieldwork coordinator, clients at the fieldwork site, officials at the university, the student health counselor, Margaret's parents, her sex partner's family, the public relations office of the university, testing site personnel, and health insurance personnel. Are there more?

What Other Information Is Needed?

The players do not function in isolation; therefore, more information is needed regarding the interrelationships of the people and their community. For example, although Margaret is monogamous, is her sex partner monogamous? What is the current level of understanding of all the players concerning HIV? What are the policies of the university and the fieldwork site regarding infection control and Universal Precautions? Why is there concern about graduation? What is the nature of Margaret's relationship with her family, leading to her fear of discussing the issue with them? How may religious beliefs play a part in the decision-making process? What other facts would you like?

Some global questions that come to mind when analyzing this case are: Do some people experience moral conflicts or prejudices when the terms *HIV, AIDS, premarital sex,* and *client care* are juxtaposed? What does practicing safer sex imply about an individual's level of responsibility? What concerns does the public have regarding healthcare practitioners and communicable diseases?

Margaret is a student practicing monogamous safer sex who thinks she may be infected with HIV. Does she need testing? Does she need counseling? Does she need support? What are the roles and responsibilities of the fieldwork coordinator, the university, and Margaret? With so many questions and concerns, what is the actual dilemma here?

What Actions May Be Taken and What Are the Possible Consequences?

Mary Evenson is correct to discuss the facts and fiction about HIV while she analyzes this case scenario. As she points out, there is a major difference between being exposed to HIV and actually manifesting AIDS. Even though a person may test positive for HIV, full-blown symptoms may not develop until years after exposure. In any event, all healthcare personnel should adhere to strict Universal Precautions when treating clients.

This case focuses on the needs and concerns of the student. An individual could argue that having Margaret continue her fieldwork experience poses no immediate threat to clients; however, some clinical practices in occupational therapy require practitioners to come in contact with body fluids. An example is splinting clients who have injuries such as burns, open wounds, and skin disorders. In some activity groups, clients might be injured, which may lead to the possibility of exchanging body fluids with the practitioner. A brief list of such activities includes cooking, woodworking, gardening, and competitive games, in which clients might injure themselves on equipment or might slip and fall.

One option in this dilemma would be to allow Margaret to proceed with her fieldwork placement but to limit her job duties until the results of the HIV test are known. During this time, she could avoid activities such as those listed previously, thereby providing minimal risk to clients. Margaret might view this option as discriminatory, however.

An ethical answer that would be satisfactory to all of the players must be determined. Milliken and Greenblatt (1988) note that the criteria for developing strategies for dealing with the HIV include the following:

1. Goals must be ethical.
2. Methods must meet stated goals and be appropriate.
3. Policies must avoid discrimination and be justly administered.
4. Potential risks and benefits to society must be clearly identified and understood.
5. The weight of policies must fall toward benefits, not toward harm.

In Margaret's scenario, university administrators are worried about possible media attention. Who is addressing Margaret's needs? It is not unusual for students to change their fieldwork placements for many reasons. If Margaret were to change her placement, her confidentiality could be protected, and the university and clinical communities would not need to know why the change was made. The occupational therapy faculty may wish to review the *AOTA Position Statement on Occupational Therapy's Commitment to Nondiscrimination and Inclusion* (AOTA, 1999a). It notes that inclusion is based on allowing individuals to fully participate in the naturally occurring activities of society and professional organizations. The document further states that professionals are entitled to the maximum opportunities to develop and use their abilities. Limiting Margaret may go against the profession's stated position.

What about Margaret's prospective employers? The duty of the university is governed by the student's willingness to share information. According to FERPA, Margaret may tell the university she does not wish for information in her file to be released. Employers may only examine a prospective employee's skills and abilities and ask whether they can do the job. After gathering all of the facts and developing a support network, Margaret should be truthful with her employer if she is found to be HIV positive. If she later develops overt symptoms of AIDS, however, she may wish to take a job in which she will not come into direct contact with clients, such as quality improvement or staff education.

Conclusion

The case previously discussed offers the reader many options for in-depth discussions about prejudices and misconceptions that can influence actions and policies. Readers may also wish to discuss AOTA's HIV position paper (AOTA, 1989a).

Study Questions

1. What are the legal and ethical responsibilities of occupational therapy students who have HIV-positive status concerning relationships with other students, clients, and their academic program?

2. What rights do students have concerning confidentiality of HIV status and by what authority?

3. What are Universal Precautions, and how is their use implied in the AOTA Occupational Therapy Code of Ethics?

4. What moral and legal principles need to be considered in disclosing information about a practitioner's or a student's HIV status? To whom and under what conditions would this information be disclosed? What strategy did you use in making this decision?

5. Describe a clinical procedure that an occupational therapy practitioner with HIV-positive status would be considered "not otherwise qualified to perform."

The Clinician

In Chapter 5, Thomas Gutheil explains the roles of the client record and suggests strategies for successful documentation. He makes clear the dangers of false representation and the advantages of a risk management approach. The principle of beneficence, or acting in ways to promote the welfare of other people, applies to this discussion. As demonstrated, battles for more or better services are best worked out not in the patient record but in other institutional arenas. Ultimately, a practitioner's actions will be judged by what is in the written record, not by what he or she believed was right or good in a particular circumstance.

Jim Hinojosa's and Sally Poole's discussion of modalities and the domain of practice in Chapter 6 addresses questions of both ethical and legal concern. The principle of nonmaleficence dictates that practitioners act in ways that do not cause needless harm or injury to their clients. Furthermore, occupational therapists are legally bound to follow licensing laws and what is considered "reasonable and accepted" practice. In Chapter 6, the role of the occupational therapy practitioner is clarified by examining practice and licensure documents that provide the parameters of acceptable actions.

In Chapter 7, Scott Trudeau fully explains the Omnibus Budget Reconciliation Act, known as OBRA. The reader is faced with a dilemma concerning the rights of a family versus the rights of an individual family member who may be bound for a nursing home. One of the ethical principles that protects the right to autonomy for nursing home residents is that rational people have the right to be self-determining. This bears a direct relationship to the inappropriate use of restraints and the involvement of nursing home residents in their own care—the main points of discussion in this chapter.

In Chapter 8, Nina Fieldsteel addresses issues concerning confidentiality in therapy groups and support groups. What are the legal and ethical considerations for the members, group leaders, agency, and associated professionals? Occupational therapy practitioners have a primary role in using groups for intervention, prevention, management, education, and support. This chapter reveals the role of the professional in addressing ethical dilemmas in regard to the structure of the group and events of the group. The discussion is also applicable to student and manager roles as they relate to confidentiality in a group.

In all four chapters, the practitioner is faced with constraints. Yet, by following prevailing written guidelines, it is hoped that quality and uniform care can be provided with appropriate involvement of those receiving occupational therapy services.

Chapter 5

Functions of the Client Record

CASE 1: Documentation for Reimbursement

CASE 2: Insurance Dictating Treatment

CASE 3: Note Signing

with commentaries by **Thomas G. Gutheil, MD,** *and* **Penny Kyler, MA, OTR, FAOTA**

Key Terms

Compensation

Comprehensible

Continuity

Coordination

Countersigning

Vicarious liability

CASE 1: Documentation for Reimbursement

José Ramirez, an experienced occupational therapist, has just started working for a private agency. Mr. Ogden, an elderly man who has suffered a cerebral vascular accident, has been referred for services. Mr. Ramirez's employer says that Mr. Ogden should receive occupational therapy twice daily for 30-minute sessions.

After evaluating Mr. Ogden, Mr. Ramirez tells his employer that the client needs only one treatment per day. The employer tells Mr. Ramirez to do as he wishes regarding the number of daily treatments provided, but that he must document two daily treatments because that is the reimbursement allowed by Mr. Ogden's insurance carrier for his condition. Mr. Ramirez has heard from other colleagues that they lost their jobs when they did not document as requested by their employers. Knowing that, he is afraid he will lose his job if he refuses to do as his employer says.

CASE 2: Insurance Dictating Treatment

Gary Bernstein, OTR, has been treating Mrs. Jaycynski for eight weeks in the rehabilitation department of a large rehabilitation facility. Mrs. Jaycynski has made remarkable progress from her cerebrovascular accident but appears to have reached a plateau for the moment. Mr. Bernstein has eight years of experience working with clients with conditions such as Mrs. Jaycynski's and is sure that she will make more progress in therapy in another week or so.

Mrs. Jaycynski's insurance company states in the policy that if no progress can be shown at the end of each week, therapy will no longer be paid for and should cease. Mr. Bernstein is tempted to document continued progress for this week so that reimbursement will continue, even though this is not strictly true. Once reimbursement has terminated for a condition/illness, it cannot easily be restarted. Mr. Bernstein would like Mrs. Jaycynski to have the opportunity to receive occupational therapy in the next two to three weeks because he is sure she will improve more.

Is Mr. Bernstein justified in falsifying this week's progress note in the client's chart?

CASE 3: Note Signing

A large rehabilitation facility employs several certified occupational therapy assistants in their occupational therapy department. The assistants receive appropriate supervision and provide a great deal of valuable treatment; however, some clients' insurance companies will not pay for treatment provided by assistants. In these instances, the supervising occupational therapists sign off on the notes and treatment plan. The practice is known and endorsed by the facility administrators.

Occupational therapist, Marie Lipinsky, is occasionally so busy that she does not have time to get to know her assistants' clients (after Ms. Lipinsky has performed the initial evaluation) but feels confident that the highly experienced assistant is carrying out the treatment plan adequately. On these occasions, she signs off on Mr. Dubois' notes, as usual.

Is this acceptable practice?

One day, one of Mr. Dubois' clients is unhappy with the care he has received at the facility and names Ms. Lipinsky (as the supervisor) in a formal complaint filed with the administration. Mr. Dubois has carried out most of the client's treatment, but Ms. Lipinsky has signed all of the notes, as per the usual practice and the orders of the administration.

Is Ms. Lipinsky responsible for defending the treatment procedures, even though she did not carry them out? Is Ms. Lipinsky accountable for the treatment, even though she did not provide it?

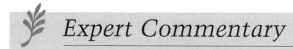

Expert Commentary

By Thomas G. Gutheil, MD

A famous cartoon shows an emergency room scene in which the doctor, with an expression of commiseration on his face, says to the grieving spouse before him: "We did all we could, but the paperwork was too much!"

This cartoon always strikes a nerve. Most practitioners in their daily work are on the brink: just a bit more paperwork and the saturation point will be reached. This regrettable state of affairs may not be able to be improved, but some aspects can become more benign with the knowledge of a few useful principles; those same principles offer considerable protection in a liability context and thus serve a risk management function as well as a record-keeping function.

What are the record-keeping functions? This chapter addresses the varying uses to which the client record is put and some strategies of successful documentation.

The Roles of the Record

Although it should go without saying, the primary role of the record is to permit client care to proceed in a continuous, coordinated, comprehensible, and, in some cases, compensable manner.

Continuity relates to the fact that client care may take place over varying time periods. To keep track of a treatment program that may extend over years and through several caretakers, the record serves as an archive of the developing care on a continuous basis.

Especially with a multidisciplinary team—a common treatment modality today—it remains essential that all care providers "push the same way." That is, they should *coordinate* their efforts so that they work synergistically and not at cross purposes. The record permits pooling of information over time by different care providers, who are able to review each other's work and to dovetail their own contributions into the plan of treatment.

The best treatment is empirical; that is, treatment evolves, in concert with

Box 5-1 *Summary*

The record-keeping standard of **continuity** refers to the fact that client care may take place over a long period with several caretakers. The record serves as an archive throughout the period of care.

Box 5-2 *Summary*

A second standard related to record-keeping, **coordination,** means that all care providers move in the same direction with the client. The record permits sharing and coordination of information.

assessments and evaluations on the basis of what works and what doesn't. To permit the kind of overview that renders long and complex treatment *comprehensible,* the record contains and concentrates the data for review, reminder, and, in some contexts research (Box 5-3).

Finally, the record permits accountability for work done and for care omitted, for *compensation* by third-party payors, utilization review, and, in the worst instance, defense against charges of malpractice (Box 5-4).

Box 5-3 *Summary*

The third standard is that the record should make long and complex treatment **comprehensible.**

Box 5-4 *Summary*

Finally, the record provides accountability for work done (and omitted) for **compensation** by third-party payors, utilization review, and sometimes as a defense against charges of malpractice.

Approaches to Documentation

Documentation is so burdensome at times that it would try the patience of most professionals to be told to "write more"; in fact, such advice is not useful and perhaps even harmful. Most clinicians are "written out" already and, curiously, merely writing more does not produce a superior record from either clinical or risk management viewpoints (Box 5-5).

Instead of writing more, write smarter. This means practitioners actually write less than they may have thought necessary because they are writing with greater efficiency. This efficiency is achieved by understanding the employment of three essential principles of documentation: (1) risk-benefit analysis, (2) exercise of clinical judgment at decision points, and (3) the client's capacity to contribute. These same principles prove to be the linchpins of good clinical care. Hence, like all good risk management concepts, this one rests solidly on a sound clinical foundation (Box 5-6).

Box 5-5 *Summary*

Merely "writing more" does not produce a superior record from either a clinical or a risk management point of view.

Box 5-6 *Summary*

Three essential principles of documentation provide the linchpins of good clinical care:

1. Risk-benefit analysis
2. Exercise of clinical judgment at decision points
3. Client's capacity to contribute

Risk-Benefit Analysis

The first principle is to document, however it is described, a risk-benefit analysis. Picture a decision tree with different forks indicating the choices or directions in which therapy may proceed. These forks often represent the "yes" or "no" of a single decision. For example, this might take the form: "Start sheltered workshop" versus "Do *not* start sheltered workshop," or "Permit sharps to be used" versus "Do not permit sharps to be used," and so on. *Each* of the two choices, yes or no, has certain risks and certain benefits. Although the risks of yes may simply be the benefits of no, many clinical situations are sufficiently complex that this simple symmetry does not apply and more detailed discussion is required.

The appearance of a risk-benefit discussion in a record accomplishes several valuable goals: (1) it reveals care in planning and consideration for the client's welfare; (2) it refutes the charge of negligence in planning, which might be part of a malpractice action; and (3) it justifies the final decision for reimbursement and utilization review purposes.

Exercise of Clinical Judgment at Decision Points

One of the most heartbreaking things to read in a record whose author has been accused of malpractice is an entry such as "Patient still bleeding. (Signed) J. Smith, M.D." The dazzling acumen of this observation is completely eclipsed by the apparent absence of any response! It makes a person want to say, "Nice pickup, Doctor Wizard, but is there anything you would like to *do* about it? Such as stop the bleeding?"

The issue here is clinical judgment, which can be formally dissected into assessment and response: What did the practitioner do, based on what he or she saw? As before, such data in the record both defend and justify one's clinical decision-making process for the various purposes already noted. Less obviously, the clinician derives the benefit from being the person who was the only observer on the scene at the time. This unique perspective appropriately defeats the clinician's having his or her judgment criticized by subsequent second guessing, but only if the incident was recorded.

Client's Capacity to Contribute

One quality that practitioners often evaluate, but may not document in these terms, is the client's capacity or ability (a form of competence) to participate in his or her own care. This includes not only the client's ability to be somewhat self-monitoring and self-regulating, but also the ability to report on inner states such as psychotic confusion or suicidal tendencies. The client who manifests this capacity may be delegated significant responsibility for various aspects of the therapy process; less intensive monitoring may be acceptable and, in case of a bad outcome, defensible.

Documentation that focuses on these three principles can be crisp while simultaneously addressing the record-keeping concerns described at the outset.

Pitfalls of Documentation

The primary pitfall of documentation is both simple and discouragingly common, and the remedy, self-explanatory: Never, *ever*, change an existing record. Not only does such "fudging" suggest (or even constitute) fraud, it is the "kiss of death" in a malpractice action, even if the care is impeccable otherwise. Jurors who sense a coverup become hostile and punitive toward caretakers.

Second only to changing an existing record, in terms of self-inflicted damage to the clinicians, is the creation of false entries. This occurs when the record reports events or caretaking that did not occur (Box 5-7). This appears to be taking place in the case example of Mr. Ramirez entitled "Documentation for Reimbursement," in which Mr. Ramirez's employer pressures him to document treatments that are not occurring to permit reimbursement. Such actions are unethical and corrupt. Mr. Ramirez faces the classic whistleblower's dilemma—to comply and commit fraud or protest and risk loss of job. Although we cannot solve Mr. Ramirez's dilemma for him, we can further study the problem by asking: Suppose Mr. Ramirez goes along and reports two treatments instead of one, what harm does that do except to the insurance company in some trivial way?

> **Box 5-7 _By the Law_**
>
> NEVER change an existing record, and NEVER create false entries.

One answer is that something may go wrong with the fragile elderly client described in the case, and the determination about whether something negligent was done might depend on witnesses, such as Mr. Ramirez, during one of the fictitious treatments. One can imagine the scenario when a fall out of bed, for example, which occurred during an alleged treatment, had no witnesses!

A similar problem afflicts Mr. Bernstein in the case entitled "Insurance Dictating Treatment." Mr. Bernstein is tempted to falsify a progress note to permit continued insurance to fund a client's poststroke rehabilitation; the compensation scheme provides reimbursement only if progress is continuous, but the client has reached a plateau, although further progress is anticipated in the future. Should Mr. Bernstein claim nonexistent progress to continue funding (which, once stopped, cannot easily be restarted)?

It is tempting to manipulate the system in the service of the client's welfare in situations like this one, especially when the insurance company's policies appear to be irrational and not relevant to the vicissitudes of clinical care; however, falsifying data is fraud. Perhaps the issue here is best viewed as a question of where to fight the battle?

Mr. Bernstein could tell the truth and donate services for a bit longer or arrange for indigent care from another agency. The fight, as it were, should not be fought in the client's record but at the agency level. For example, healthcare organizations may exert pressure on carriers or legislative action may require adjustment to the realities of recovery from stroke. Fighting the battle in the record, in contrast, may harm both client and practitioner.

Signatures and Record-Keeping

A practitioner's signature at the bottom of a note is usually unambiguous: he or she signed it because he or she wrote it. With countersignature, the matter becomes more complex. Countersigning, depending on context and policy, may mean anything from "I have read this note" to "I approve of this note's content" (plan, observations, and so on) to "I have reviewed this therapy in a supervisory capacity" to "I take ultimate responsibility for the care here rendered and recorded" and so on. Such ambiguity is not only confusing, but it is also dangerous in a liability context.

The underlying risk management concept here is *vicarious liability,* a term referring to the way in which an individual may be liable for the actions of another, usually but not always a junior, an employee, or a subordinate (Box 5-8).

The connection between vicarious liability and signatures is best captured in the risk management axiom, "If you sign, the case is thine." Countersignature of a treatment plan, insurance form, prescription for medication, progress note, or similar document is usually tantamount to declaring oneself responsible, vicariously, for the treatment in question. In a malpractice action, consequently, signing off on the occasions previously noted constitutes signing on as a defendant (Box 5-9).

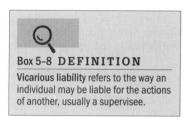

Box 5-8 DEFINITION

Vicarious liability refers to the way an individual may be liable for the actions of another, usually a supervisee.

Box 5-9 *By the Law*

Countersigning treatment plans and notes in a client's record usually means the signer is taking on responsibility for the client.

Turning now to the case example of Mr. Dubois and Ms. Lipinsky, entitled "Note Signing," note that supervising therapist Ms. Lipinsky signs off on assistant Mr. Dubois' notes even on such occasions when she does not get to know Mr. Dubois' clients. Because the example reports that Ms. Lipinsky "feels confident that the highly experienced assistant is carrying out the treatment plan adequately," this action is defensible as an act of delegation. The clients, however, are still Ms. Lipinsky's responsibility.

The answers to the queries posed in the example become evident from the foregoing discussion. Ms. Lipinsky is responsible for defending the treatment procedures even though she did not carry them out. Hence, Ms. Lipinsky is legitimately a target of a formal complaint or of litigation. In other words, Ms. Lipinsky is accountable.

A surprising number of professionals are unaware of their vicarious responsibilities for those with whom they work. When in doubt, prudent

Box 5-10 *Summary*

If practitioners have supervisees assigned to them, they have a responsibility to "credential" the trainees.

professionals define, as early as possible in employment, for whom they are responsible. If practitioners have supervisees or employees assigned to them, they have the burden of either "credentialing" the trainees (as Ms. Lipinsky has apparently done with Mr. Dubois) or supervising them frequently enough that they are on top of the cases. The more capable trainees are, the lighter may be the supervisory touch, but the determination of how much scrutiny supervisees require must be made on an individual basis; it is hazardous to assume skills without evidence (Box 5-10).

Conclusion

The record's primary function remains that of documenting and facilitating clinical care. Over and above that purpose, the principles previously noted will not only aid in realizing the clinical goal but will also prove valuable in risk management.

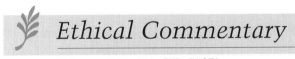

Ethical Commentary

By Penny Kyler, MA, OTR, FAOTA

Some of the terms relevant to the case of Mr. Ramirez and Mr. Ogden and the case of Ms. Lipinsky and Mr. Dubois are *whistleblowing, fraud, falsifying data, vicarious liability,* and *competence.* These terms raise considerable anxiety in most circles. In health care, the temptation to engage in fraud by falsifying records may have increased because of recent heightened pressure to produce billable treatments. Add-itionally, the rush to see more individuals and the assumption that another colleague is competent and will follow treatment plans may have compromised Ms. Lipinsky (Box 5-11).

Box 5-11 *Summary*

The temptation to engage in fraud by falsifying records has increased because of heightened pressure to produce billable treatments.

Case 1: Documentation for Reimbursement

The dilemma Mr. Ramirez faces is one that may confront other occupational therapy practitioners today. More and more frequently, insurers and utilization review groups seem to be dictating practice, although, in the case of Mr. Ramirez, the employer is asking the therapist to override the dictates of the insurance carrier. Mr. Ramirez's case is complex in that it involves the interrelationships of legal, ethical, and social problems.

Who Are the Players?

José Ramirez, the private agency, Mr. Ogden, his family, Mr. Ramirez's boss, the insurance company, the agency head, other occupational therapy staff, and other clients are the players. Are there any others?

What Other Information Is Needed?

During the initial treatment session, did Mr. Ramirez get informed consent from Mr. Ogden and did he discuss the type, duration, and frequency of treatment with him? What are the insurance guidelines set out by Mr. Ogden's insurance carrier? What is Mr. Ogden's course of progress likely to be? Has Mr. Ogden been made aware of the parameters of his insurance reimbursement? Does Mr. Ogden have an understanding of his options? Is Mr. Ogden likely to move on to home health care following his care at this agency? If so, how soon? Are other clients on a waiting list at this agency? What type of relationship does Mr. Ramirez have with his boss? To whom does his boss answer? Is there anyone else in the agency to whom Mr. Ramirez can turn for advice? Who actually is giving the order to document—his boss or the private agency? Does it make a difference if it is an individual or an entity? Do you need other information?

What Actions May Be Taken and What Are the Possible Consequences?

The legal issue here is fraud, either for documentation of services not rendered or for providing more services than are clinically indicated. *Fraud*, as defined by Gifis (1984), is making a false representation with an evil intent. Although Mr. Ramirez is obviously uncomfortable about this situation, if he was to give in and document services that he had not provided or to give more treatment than he thought was necessary, he would be making false representation—committing fraud.

Occupational therapy practitioners in licensed states are at risk of losing their licenses if they commit fraud. Fraud is also an overt breach of the AOTA Code of Ethics (2000a), which in several places addresses the dilemmas identified in this case. These include, Principle I.B: "The individual shall establish fees, based on cost analysis, that are commensurate with services rendered." Principle 3.A: "Occupational therapy practitioners shall collaborate with service recipients in setting goals and priorities during the intervention process." Principle 5.A: "The individual shall be acquainted with applicable local, state, federal, and institutional rules and Association policies and shall function accordingly."

Principles 5.B: "The individual shall inform employers, employees and colleagues about those laws and policies that apply to the profession of occupational therapy," and 5.D: "Occupational therapy practitioners shall take reasonable steps to ensure employers are aware of occupational therapy's ethical obligations."

It is undoubtedly income for the agency that is motivating the employer to push Mr. Ramirez into excess treatment sessions. Mr. Ramirez could attempt to take the moral high road with his employer by discussing the ethical and legal implications of the employer's demands. He could also suggest that he be allowed to generate additional income for the agency by adding another client to his caseload during the second time period allotted for Mr. Ogden. On the other hand, Mr. Ramirez could discuss with Mr. Ogden his progress in relation to the requirements of his insurance carrier, thereby making him an informed participant in decisions concerning his treatment. Mr. Ramirez would be behaving ethically by allowing the client to exercise autonomy, in accordance with the AOTA Code of Ethics, Principles 3.A and 3.D: "The individual shall collaborate with those people served in the treatment planning process and respect the right of the individual to refuse treatment."

Fear, although an uncomfortable emotion, should not be used as an excuse for not acting in the best interests of the profession, the client, or one's personal beliefs. There are laws that protect whistleblowers. It should also be noted that the costs for falsifying claims sent to insurance companies are ultimately passed on to consumers. Inherent in the obligations of being occupational therapy practitioners are the obligations healthcare providers have to provide for the welfare of society—called *social justice* in ethics terms. Mr. Ramirez is a member of a greater community of healthcare providers and must weigh the needs of the many against the needs of the few. Whose need is of greater importance? How does Mr. Ramirez's professional obligation fit into the total picture?

When a relationship between an occupational therapy practitioner and a client is formed, it is presumed to be therapeutic. At a minimum, the practitioner is expected to practice competently and not to harm the client through acts of omission or commission—in other words, to practice with fidelity or faithfulness. Acting with fidelity is a type of promise-keeping that focuses practitioners on their obligations to the profession and to their clients. Mr. Ramirez has a duty to act with fidelity toward his client, Mr. Ogden.

Mr. Ramirez could choose to function within the boundaries of ethics that focus on moral obligations, commitment, and duties. Following this approach, Mr. Ramirez would choose his course of action based on his obligations. His decision would focus not only on the consequences of his actions but also on what he perceives as his binding duty. Mr. Ramirez has duties by virtue of being an occupational therapist interacting with a more vulnerable human being. He also has a duty by virtue of his role as an individual within a greater community. Some actions he might choose, if he were to practice from a deontologic point of view, would be to feel obligated to go over his boss's head and report the potential fraud or to ignore his boss and document only those treatments given.

Case 3: Note Signing

In Ms. Lipinsky and Mr. Dubois' scenario, they should be concerned with a possible breach of the AOTA Code of Ethics, Principle 5.C: "The individual who employs or supervises colleagues shall provide appropriate supervision, as defined in AOTA guidelines or state laws, regulations, and institutional policies" (AOTA, 2000a).

Who Are the Players?

Ms. Lipinsky, Mr. Dubois, the administrator, the clients, the lawyers, the insurance company, and the other staff are the players. Are there other players?

What Other Information Is Needed?

What is the specific nature of the complaint? Is it defensible? Has something illegal or unethical occurred? What is the role of the hospital administrator? What do the other staff members think? What policies and procedures are in place defining the roles, functions, and supervision of occupational therapists and occupational therapy assistants? What are the prevailing community practice standards? Is this a state in which occupational therapists and/or occupational therapy assistants are licensed? If so, what does the practice act say about signing off on an occupational therapy assistant's records? Are other facts needed to analyze this case?

What Actions May Be Taken and What Are the Possible Consequences?

In Dr. Gutheil's commentary, he is correct in noting that prudent professionals provide supervision with sufficient frequency that the supervisor is kept abreast of the supervisee's cases. This comment is consistent with the AOTA's perspective on supervision. It is of concern that Ms. Lipinsky was so busy that she did not have time to properly supervise Mr. Dubois and that she was unfamiliar with his clients. It is generally accepted within the profession that occupational therapists and occupational therapy assistants function as a team and that they collaborate. The collaboration between Ms. Lipinsky and Mr. Dubois had broken down. The role and scope of practice for each level of occupational therapy practitioner are outlined by the AOTA in a document entitled "Occupational Therapy Roles" (1993b) and in state practice acts. In both cases, adequate supervision of assistants by occupational therapists is described and decreed. The key phrase in the paper on occupational therapy roles is that "The level of supervision is related to the ability of the COTA to safely and effectively provide those interventions delegated by an OTR" (p. 1090). Principle 4.B of the AOTA Code of Ethics indicates that practitioners "should conform to standards of practice and other appropriate AOTA documents relevant to practice" (p.615).

According to nurses Curtin and Flaherty (1999), a person's professional prerogative includes the right to receive support, correction, and guidance from one's colleagues. When the caseload became so great that Ms. Lipinsky had little time to get to know her assistant's clients, she should have exercised her professional responsibility of limiting her caseload. Additionally, Ms. Lipinsky should be guided by the AOTA Code of Ethics (2000a) and the Guidelines to the Code of Ethics (1998b). The prudent practitioner would note that she has a responsibility, not only to her profession, but also to her clients, her employer, and her colleagues.

Study Questions

1. What is the function of the client record?

2. What is the value of including a risk-benefit analysis in documentation?

3. What things should an occupational therapy practitioner never do in documentation?

4. Why is it wise for the practitioner to include clients in planning and locating appropriate reimbursement for their treatment programs? What legal and ethical dilemmas may be avoided by such an approach?

5. What is the highest authority dictating the content of documentation?

Modalities and Domain of Practice

CASE: Ultrasound Intervention

with commentaries by **Jim Hinojosa, PhD, OT, FAOTA; Sally Poole, MA, OT, CHT;** *and* **Penny Kyler, MA, OTR, FAOTA**

Key Terms

Conduction
Convection
Conversion
Domain of concern

Frame of reference
Physical agent modalities
Thermal modalities
Tools

CASE: Ultrasound Intervention

Tony Murphy is a recent graduate of an entry-level master's program in occupational therapy. He considers himself lucky to have been offered a staff occupational therapy position at a major teaching hospital, where he has the opportunity to rotate through a variety of services. His first rotation is in the outpatient occupational therapy clinic, where persons with hand, orthopedic, and sports injuries are treated. He works in the clinic with one other experienced supervising occupational therapist.

Mr. Murphy received his undergraduate degree in psychology. He had completed several volunteer experiences throughout his college years to help him decide on a career path. He volunteered in a variety of occupational therapy settings but was most fascinated by occupational therapy in a local hand clinic, where he saw a variety of hand and upper quadrant injuries, including work-related injuries, sports injuries, repetitive stress syndrome, and trauma. He was somewhat disappointed that his occupational therapy education did not devote much classroom time to this area, but he completed level I fieldwork in a hand clinic.

Mr. Murphy has now been on the job for two months, and today is the first day that he is working alone because his supervising therapist is ill. He must see the new client who was originally scheduled to be evaluated and treated by his supervisor. The new client, Ms. Sonderheim, is referred by an orthopedist with the diagnosis of bilateral lateral epicondylitis. The referral asks for a comprehensive occupational therapy evaluation and treatment to include ultrasound, soft tissue mobilization, range of motion, and ergonomic instruction to prevent a reoccurrence.

Mr. Murphy completes the initial evaluation and gives the client a home program. Because she is in pain, he wants to begin treatment today but has not as yet used the ultrasound machine. He sees that it is not a unit with which he is familiar and is not sure of the parameters of the machine. Ms. Sonderheim demands that the physician's orders be followed to the letter; she has had lateral epicondylitis before and finds that ultrasound is extremely helpful in pain reduction. Mr. Murphy reads the instruction manual for the ultrasound machine quickly and applies ultrasound as ordered by the physician. Ms. Sonderheim complains of pain during the treatment, but Mr. Murphy assures her that it will take only a "few more minutes."

The next day, Mr. Murphy is summoned by the supervising occupational therapist, who wants to know what happened with Ms. Sonderheim. Apparently, one day after the ultrasound treatment, the client called her doctor with complaints of redness, swelling, and increased pain in both elbows. The physician then called the supervisor complaining about the treatment his client received. The supervising occupational therapist is furious because she found the ultrasound machine set on "uninterrupted mode" (i.e., direct mode, which could harm a client). She asks Mr. Murphy for an explanation.

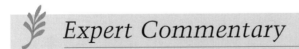

Expert Commentary

By Jim Hinojosa, PhD, OT, FAOTA, and Sally Poole, MA, OT, CHT

Introduction

Therapeutic modalities and other legitimate tools of a profession change over time in response to the knowledge and skills of practitioners, advances in technology, changes in society, and the needs and values of the profession (Luebben, Hinojosa, & Kramer, 1999) (Boxes 6-1, 6-2). Changes and shifts in the modalities and tools used by practitioners

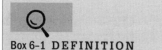

Box 6-1 DEFINITION

Thermal modalities are methods of heat transfer that include conduction, convection, and conversion. **Conduction** is the transfer of heat between two parts caused by a temperature difference between the parts; **convection** is the transfer of heat by the circulation of heated parts of a liquid or gas; and **conversion** is the transformation from one material or state to another. All thermal modalities fall into one of these three categories.

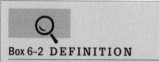

Box 6-2 DEFINITION

Tools are the items, means, methods, and instruments that are used in practice in a theoretically proscribed manner to bring about change (Mosey, 1986).

Box 6-3 DEFINITION

Physical agent modalities are therapeutic agents that "use the properties of light, water, temperature, sound, and electricity to produce a response in soft tissue" (McGuire et al., 1991, p. 6). According to AOTA's Task Force on Physical Agent Modalities, physical agents include, but are not limited to, paraffin baths, hot packs, cold packs, fluidotherapy, contrast baths, ultrasound, whirlpool baths, and electrical stimulation (McGuire et al., 1991).

guarantee that the profession remains viable and responsive to clients' and society's needs. Practitioners tend to hold the modalities and tools they use in high regard, and some believe that modalities and tools used for intervention define the scope of occupational therapy practice. Some practitioners believe that certain modalities or tools should be used by occupational therapy practitioners, whereas others believe that these same modalities or tools should not be used within occupational therapy.

In the 1980s, one of occupational therapy's controversial issues was the use of physical agent modalities by occupational therapy practitioners (Box 6-3). Some condemned the use of physical agent modalities, whereas others asserted that physical agent modalities were an important intervention tool for the profession. After an intense debate, the 1991 Representative Assembly of the American Occupational Therapy Association (AOTA) adopted the following statement:

> Physical agent modalities may be used as an adjunct to, or in preparation for purposeful activity to enhance occupational performance and when applied by a practitioner who has documented evidence of possessing the theoretical background and technical skills for safe and competent integration of the modality into an occupational therapy intervention plan.
>
> (AOTA, 1991)

Physical Agent Modalities

Physical agent modalities are defined as nonhuman physical agents that "use the properties of light, water, temperature, sound, and electricity to produce a response in soft tissue" (McGuire et al., 1991, p. 6). They include physical agents such as paraffin baths, hot packs, cold packs, fluidotherapy, contrast baths, ultrasound, whirlpool, and electrical stimulation.

Table 6–1
Effects of Heat and Cold Thermal Agents

Physical System	Heat	Cold
Blood flow	Increases	Decreases
Tissue temperature	Increases	Decreases
Tissue extensibility	Increases	Decreases
Joint stiffness	Decreases	Increases
Muscle strain/spasm	Decreases	Decreases

Occupational therapy practitioners sometimes use physical agent modalities in conjunction with or in preparation for client engagement in purposeful activity or occupation, believing that this intervention will support the individual's capacity to participate in a task or activity. Clinicians apply physical agent modalities within the context of a theoretically based guideline for interventions (i.e., a frame of reference, model, or paradigm).

The most common physical agent modalities used by occupational therapy practitioners are thermal agents (i.e., agents used to either raise or lower the temperature of soft tissue). A heat modality may be used when a therapist wants to reduce pain and stiffness and improve tissue healing, whereas heat is generally contraindicated when an increased blood flow is not wanted (e.g., with hemophilia or post-traumatic edema) or in the presence of malignancy (Bracciano & Earley, 2002; Breines, 2001; Michlovitz, 1991). Cold agent modalities (cryotherapies), on the other hand, are used to reduce acute or postexercise edema, pain, and inflammation. The use of a cold modality is contraindicated in the presence of decreased sensation or peripheral vascular disease, or after a limb or body part has been replanted (Bracciano & Earley, 2002). Table 6-1 briefly summarizes the effects of heat and cold on the physical system.

There are three methods of heat transfer: conduction, convection, and conversion. *Conduction* is the transfer of heat between two parts caused by a temperature difference between the parts; *convection* is the transfer of heat by the circulation of heated parts of a liquid or gas; and *conversion* is the transformation from one material or state to another. All thermal modalities fall into one of these three categories (Table 6-2).

This chapter discusses four issues related to the implications of the use of physical agent modalities by occupational therapy practitioners.

Do Physical Agent Modalities Fall Within The Scope of Practice of Occupational Therapy?

As occupational therapy evolves, the goals and priorities of the profession shift and change in response to social, political, informational, and

Table 6–2
Comparison of Thermal Modalities*

Method	Technique	Advantages	Disadvantages	Precautions/ Contra-indications
Conduction	Hot packs	Superficial, moist heat easy to use	No range of motion while heating	Body part should not be on top of the heating unit
	Paraffin	Low, specific heat easier to tolerate	Affected part not observable; no range of motion while heating	Not for open or infected wounds
	Cold packs	Reduce pain, spasticity	Patient intolerance	Decreased sensation: peripheral vascular disease
Convection	Whirlpool	Wound care; patient comfort; range of motion	May increase edema due to dependent position of limb	Should not to be used as heating agent only
	Fluid therapy	Range of motion while heating; less likely to increase edema	Expensive	Not for wet open wounds
Conversion	Ultrasound	Penetration of heat to deeper structures; reduces scarring; improves tendon extensibility	Excessive heating	Pacemaker; malignancy; bone/skin wound

*This table presents an overview and is not considered to be comprehensive.

technological innovations. Its ability to adapt and change in response to society's priorities, new knowledge, and technological innovation is a strength of occupational therapy. As the profession's goals and priorities change, some interventions used by practitioners also change; however, these changes should always be consistent with occupational therapy's primary focus on occupation and a person's ability to engage in occupation as a social human being (AOTA, 1979).

The domain of concern of a profession is the unique area of expertise specific to that profession (Mosey, 1986, 1996) (Box 6-4). In an effort to define occupational therapy's domain of concern and areas of expertise, several documents have been developed by the AOTA. In 1979, 1989, and 1994, the AOTA adopted taxonomies that outlined the profession's domain in terms of performance components, performance areas, and performance contexts. The most recent document to outline the domain of concern of the profession is the Occupational Therapy Practice Framework: Domain and Process (AOTA, 2002). It was "developed in response to current practice needs—the need to more clearly affirm and articulate occupational therapy's unique focus on occupation and daily life activities and the application of an intervention process that facilitates engagement in occupation to support participation in life" (p. 1). The purpose of the document is: "(a) to describe the domain that centers and grounds the profession's focus and action and (b) to outline the process of occupational therapy evaluation and intervention that is dynamic and linked to the profession's focus on and use of occupation" (p. 1).

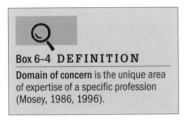

Box 6-4 **DEFINITION**

Domain of concern is the unique area of expertise of a specific profession (Mosey, 1986, 1996).

According to the Practice Framework, the expertise of occupational therapy practitioners is in their ability to facilitate a client's engagement in occupation to support the individual's participation in his or her own context. A practitioner attends to context, activity demands, and client factors to influence the individual's performance skills and patterns (AOTA, 2002). In addition, the practitioner intervenes to address the client's motor performance skill deficits by examining factors within and outside the individual that influence his or her skill performance. During occupational therapy intervention, "the focus remains on occupation, and efforts are directed toward fostering improved engagement in an occupation or occupations. A variety of therapeutic activities, including engagement in actual daily life activities and occupations, are used in intervention" (p. 13). The important point for this chapter is that physical agent modalities are often used as preparatory or facilitating methods, to prepare a client for performance in areas of occupation.

Individual practitioners determine what tools or modalities they will use that are consistent with their beliefs about the profession, their knowledge and skills, and the needs of the clients. Fundamentally, there are two conflicting perspectives on whether occupational therapy practitioners should use physical agent modalities or not. Practitioners who oppose the use of physical agent modalities base their interpretation on the basic philosophy of occupational therapy (Fidler, 1992). They support the use of purposeful activities, occupation, and the traditional creative and manual arts. They view physical agent modalities as passive in nature, as doing something *to* an individual. The use of interventions that are passive do not fit in with their conviction that occupational therapy must involve the client in an *active* process. Furthermore, they believe that physical agent modalities fall within the domain of concern of physical therapy and are concerned about the implications of duplication of interventions by the two professions.

Other therapists support the use of physical agent modalities in conjunction with or to facilitate a client's ability to engage in purposeful activity or occupation. They agree that physical agent modalities are passive but argue that occupational therapy practitioners often use tools that allow the client to develop the ability to do something or to prevent dysfunction. Splinting and some assistive devices are viewed in this way. In addition, these practitioners state explicitly that physical agent modalities are used to prepare or support the client's ability to participate or engage in occupation. Thus the use of a physical agent modality can be either facilitatory or inhibitory. The authors of this chapter support this perspective. Furthermore, the authors believe that any occupational therapy intervention must be developed and applied within the context of a frame of reference that will organize theoretical information so that it can be applied therapeutically (Mosey, 1970, 1986, 1996) (Box 6-5).

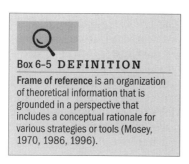

Box 6-5 DEFINITION

Frame of reference is an organization of theoretical information that is grounded in a perspective that includes a conceptual rationale for various strategies or tools (Mosey, 1970, 1986, 1996).

The application of any frame of reference involves the use of a variety of intervention strategies and tools. Tools are the items, means, methods, and instruments that are used for intervention in a theoretically proscribed manner to bring about change. Occupational therapy practitioners use a variety of tools, including interpersonal processes (such as conscious use of self and group work), activity processes (such as elements of performance areas and stimulus-response activities), and physical modalities (such as physical agents, atmospheric elements, and technological products) (Mosey, 1996).

As mentioned earlier, some practitioners hold the profession's tools and modalities in high regard and may even consider them to be symbolic of the profession as a whole (Kramer & Hinojosa, 1993). In reality, however, the tools and modalities used by occupational therapy practitioners are not unique and are shared by many professions. For example, nurses, physicians, and physical therapists commonly use physical agent modalities, whereas educators, psychologists, and recreation therapists use purposeful activities. A profession does not own its tools. Occupational therapy does not own purposeful activities nor does physical therapy own physical agent modalities.

Do Occupational Therapy Practitioners Have The Educational Background to Support The Use of Physical Agent Modalities?

Upon entry into any healthcare profession, a practitioner cannot know everything that is necessary to provide appropriate intervention in every situation. Furthermore, entry-level education is general in nature and does not prepare the practitioner for specialty areas of practice.

Every accredited program for occupational therapists and occupational therapy assistants in the United States must be in compliance with the Standards for an Accredited Educational Program for the Occupational Therapist and for the Occupational Therapy Assistant (Accreditation Council for Occupational Therapy [ACOTE], 1999a, 1999b). These standards set minimum requirements that must be included in an educational curriculum for entry-level occupational therapy practitioners. They outline general areas of content but do not specify explicit content, specific courses, or particular intervention strategies. Each professional educational program must configure a curriculum that meets the intent and content outlined in the Standards, and any curriculum can include content or information beyond the minimum requirements set by the Standards. AOTA's official position is that the use of physical agent modalities is not considered entry-level practice (AOTA, 1997); therefore, expertise in their use is not mentioned in the Standards.

Along with many other tools of the profession, physical agent modalities are not mandated or described in the Standards; however, the foundations on which these modalities are based are included: anatomy, kinesiology, physiology, and the neurosciences. The Standards consist of an outline of the minimum base of knowledge needed to begin practicing in the profession of occupational therapy. In 1999, the AOTA adopted Standards for Continuing Competence (AOTA, 1999b) to assist occupational therapy practitioners to assess, maintain, and document competence in all of the responsibilities and roles they assume. Continuing competence is the responsibility of the individual practitioner. It is a dynamic, multidimensional process that ensures that the practitioner has the knowledge, performance skills, interpersonal abilities, critical reasoning skills, and ethical reasoning skills needed for his or her practice.

It is generally accepted that the knowledge and skills learned in basic professional education are not adequate for the safe and effective use of physical agent modalities. Ultimately, it is the practitioner's responsibility to obtain training for use of any tool that he or she chooses to use. Accordingly, a practitioner who chooses to use physical agent modalities must get appropriate educational training beyond basic professional education. For some practitioners, basic information about physical agent modalities was included in their basic professional education. For others, all knowledge and skills must be obtained in postprofessional education.

Other knowledge areas considered important for the use of some physical agent modalities are physics and chemistry. Only a few accredited occupational therapy programs include physics and chemistry as part of the course of study (McGuire et al., 1991), although some practitioners may obtain knowledge in physics and chemistry in other ways.

As with any tool or modality, the competent use of physical agent modalities is not limited to technical expertise, but must also include theoretical knowledge. During fieldwork, in which students begin to provide occupational therapy under close supervision, it is not sufficient to simply learn and practice the techniques to use a physical agent modality. For example, it is necessary to know not only how to apply a hot pack but also how the treatment relates to the specific injury, its effects on the specific tissues involved, and its impact on the functional needs and requirements of the client. For the fieldwork student who is learning to use a physical agent modality, both the clinical supervisor and the student are responsible to ensure that adequate technical as well as theoretical information is provided.

The case scenario states that Mr. Murphy has had only level I fieldwork experience with physical agent modalities. Clearly, this background was insufficient for him to be considered to have the theoretical and technical expertise to use ultrasound as a therapeutic intervention.

When are Occupational Therapy Practitioners Competent to Use Physical Agent Modalities?

All occupational therapy practitioners are expected to comply with the Occupational Therapy Code of Ethics (AOTA, 2000a) and the Standards for Continuing Competence (AOTA, 1999b). Of particular concern to Mr. Murphy in the scenario are Principles 3 and 4 in the Occupational Therapy Code of Ethics that specifically address areas of concern for practitioners who choose to use physical agent modalities. Principle 3 states: "Occupational therapy personnel shall respect the recipient and/or their surrogate(s) as well as the recipient's rights (autonomy, privacy, confidentiality)." Principle 3.B requires that a practitioner fully inform a client about the nature, risks, and potential outcomes of interventions. Therefore, a practitioner who plans to use physical agent modalities must inform the client about the treatment and the expected outcome. It is ultimately the client's decision whether the physical agent should be used. Finally, Principle 3.D requires that the practitioner respect the client's decision.

Of particular relevance to Mr. Murphy is Principle 4, which states, "Occupational therapy personnel shall achieve and continually maintain high standards of competence (duties)" (p.615). This principle requires that a practitioner hold appropriate credentials, follow Standards of Practice, assume responsibility for maintaining and documenting competency, and follow evidence-based research findings regarding the efficacy of physical agent modalities. This principle is expanded on in the Standards of Continuing Competence (AOTA, 1999b), requiring all members of the profession to demonstrate competent professional behavior and conduct (Hinojosa et al., 2000a, 2000b). Each practitioner is obligated to develop an individualized plan to meet his or her own competency needs.

These Standards recognize that rapid changes in technology and knowledge necessitate that a clinician engage in lifelong learning. Most important, the Standards acknowledge that an occupational therapy practitioner who uses physical agent modalities must demonstrate knowledge, performance skills, interpersonal abilities, and critical and ethical reasoning skills that embrace occupational therapy's beliefs about occupation and their impact on human performance. Ethics of professional practice are grounded in the conviction that practitioners must provide competent intervention that will have beneficial results; they must use ethical responsibility to monitor their own behaviors when it comes to the use of physical agent modalities.

When a healthcare practitioner is competent in an area of practice, society and the recipient of intervention are assured that the person providing the service has the appropriate knowledge and skills to intervene safely and effectively. An occupational therapy practitioner who is competent in the use of physical agent modalities has prerequisite knowledge and skills, possesses sufficient theoretical knowledge, and is able to determine the expected outcomes of the treatment. Theoretical and technical bodies of knowledge necessary for the safe and appropriate use of physical agent modalities are as follows:

1. Course(s) in human anatomy
2. Principles of chemistry and physics related to specific properties of light, water, temperature, sound, or electricity, as indicated by selected modalities
3. Physiological, neurophysiological, and electrophysiological changes that occur as a result of the application of selected modalities
4. The response of normal and abnormal tissue to the application of the modality
5. Indications and contraindications related to the selection and application of the modality
6. Guidelines for treatment or administration of the modality
7. Guidelines for preparing the patient, including educating the patient about the process and possible outcomes of treatment (risks and benefits)
8. Safety rules and precautions related to specific modalities
9. Methods for documenting the effectiveness of immediate and long-term effects of treatment
10. Characteristics of the equipment, including safe operation, adjustment, indications of malfunction, and care of the equipment
11. Supervised use of the physical agent modality until service competency and professional judgment in selection, modification, and integration into the occupational therapy program is ensured (McGuire et al., 1991, p. 47)

A difficulty inherent in determining someone's competence is that a professional often cannot be categorized as simply competent or incompetent. Instead, a continuum exists, with an individual being either more or less competent in the use of each specific modality. At entry into a profession, practitioners often are not competent in some specific area of practice even though they have the basic skills necessary to safely and effectively intervene with most clients. As they mature and develop advanced skills, practitioners become more confident and skilled in many areas of practice, including the use of specific modalities. Confidence and skill are influenced by clinical experience, increased body of knowledge, and an individual's life experience; with increased confidence and knowledge, the practitioner moves toward the highly competent end of the continuum. With increased competence, the practitioner is able to assess his or her effectiveness and can more easily assess the effectiveness of a tool or an intervention strategy. In essence, with competence, the practitioner becomes more artful in the use of tools and other intervention strategies.

Is It Legal for Occupational Therapy Practitioners to Use Physical Agent Modalities?

States may regulate the practice of any profession through a variety of means to protect the public from unqualified practitioners, to ensure professional conduct on the part of licensed personnel, and to ensure a certain level of mandatory entry-level competency (AOTA, 1989b). In short, state laws and regulations determine the scope of a profession's practice in that particular state. Although some state practice laws may specifically assert that physical therapists may use physical agent modalities, for example, these laws may not exclude their use by members of other professions such as occupational therapists, physicians, nurses, chiropractors, or athletic trainers. Usually state licensure laws are written in general terms and do not discuss the specifics of occupational therapy intervention such as physical agent modalities; however, a few states do have regulations that address the use of physical agent modalities. Each practitioner must investigate the licensure laws and regulations in any state in which they practice.

It is important to understand that state laws and regulations take precedence over any AOTA policies, standards, or guidelines. Furthermore, it is important to continually monitor state laws and regulations because they are constantly subject to change. The practitioner's professional obligation is to practice in compliance with state laws and regulations.

Summary

The authors view occupational therapy as an exciting, dynamic profession that is responsive to the needs of society. As technology and knowledge expand, occupational therapy practitioners select and use innovations during their interventions. Increasingly, these tools are becoming specific to certain areas of practice and require that individuals establish new competencies for their use. The fundamental position taken by this chapter's authors is that physical agent modalities fall into this category. The responsibility of occupational therapy practitioners who use physical agent modalities is to ensure that they have the appropriate theoretical and technical knowledge for safe and effective application. Also, it is their ethical responsibility to ensure that they are competent in the use of each modality they select.

Physical agent modalities are used by occupational therapy practitioners as adjuncts to or in preparation for purposeful activities that enhance occupational performance. As with any tool, focusing on physical agent modalities as an intervention exclusively would not be practicing occupational therapy; practitioners should become competent at using a wide variety of therapeutic tools. Further, they must continue to update and refine their knowledge and skills relative to research findings and technologic advances for all the tools they use. Finally, practitioners have an ethical responsibility to establish and monitor their own competency in tool use and have the professional obligation to practice in compliance with state laws and regulations.

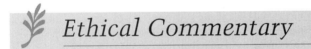

Ethical Commentary

By Penny Kyler, MA, OTR, FAOTA

Occupational therapy practitioners no longer confine their practice to using functional or purposeful activities. Some in the profession are still debating whether it is appropriate for occupational therapy practitioners to use physical agent modalities. Some have moved forward by incorporating these agents into their practices and by seeking additional certification in specialty areas. Those working in some physical disabilities settings or specialty practices such as hand surgery or orthopedics often find themselves sharing practice roles with hand therapists, physical therapists, engineers, counselors, and client advocates, as well as participating in a variety of other roles for which they were not trained in their occupational therapy program. As a profession, occupational therapy practitioners continue to debate issues surrounding the appropriate use of modalities within occupational therapy. Hinojosa and Poole have noted that physical therapists, physicians, athletic trainers, and nurses also use but do not own physical agent modalities. Those not in favor of occupational therapy practitioners using modalities note that their use carries occupational therapy away from its roots—the use of purposeful and meaningful activities.

Turning to the case, it does not state what else Mr. Murphy did with his client other than apply ultrasound; the physician had ordered a comprehensive occupational therapy evaluation and treatment to include ultrasound, soft tissue mobilization, range of motion, and ergonomic instruction to prevent a reoccurrence. But the crux of this case lies in Mr. Murphy's ability to communicate effectively to Ms. Sonderheim his level of competence and his need to be working under supervision. Sometimes one does not wish to share with the individual receiving service one's lack of training. This omission can be a critical error. It is wiser to share what one does not know and seek guidance than not to share and to do something in error. At this point, litigation by recipients of service is a possibility that must be understood not as a threat but as a fact of life. Mr. Murphy's intent was to do good; however, it appears that a quick reading of an instruction manual did not adequately prepare him to carry out the ultrasound treatment.

Who Are the Players?

The players are Mr. Murphy, Ms. Sonderheim, the orthopedic surgeon, the supervising occupational therapist, the state licensing board, the malpractice carrier, the National Board for Certification in Occupational Therapy (NBCOT), and if Mr. Murphy is a member of the AOTA, the Commission on Standards and Ethics.

What Other Information Is Needed?

What was the extent of Mr. Murphy's knowledge regarding the diagnosis and treatment of bilateral lateral epicondylitis? Was this a standing order from the orthopedist? Was the orthopedist available to be consulted during the treatment of Ms. Sonderheim? Were other practitioners around with whom Mr. Murphy could consult? What other types of supervision were available? What other modalities and activities could Mr. Murphy have used?

In examining this dilemma, the appropriate scope of practice for a new graduate who obtained employment at a major teaching hospital and who has been practicing under supervision for a couple of months needs to be considered. One must also consider the necessary knowledge, skills, and abilities for a practitioner employed in such a position. The AOTA Code of Ethics (2000a) discusses a practitioner's competence in Principle 4.E, stating that an individual shall function within the parameters of his or her competence and the standards of the profession. Mr. Murphy may have been suffering from timidity, but at what cost? Purtilo (1989) notes that professionals may feel ethical distress when they know which of several courses of action to take but are prevented from proceeding by external barriers. Did Mr. Murphy sense a barrier preventing him from making an ethical choice? It seems more likely that he knew he was in "over his head" but that he was not sure what to do about it.

The Unites States is a consumer-oriented society in which the consumer is the ultimate decision maker. Healthcare service practitioners and managers are trying to be customer friendly even when, as in this case, providing the service may be detrimental to the recipient. Principle 4.B of the Code makes practitioners aware that certain guidelines must be followed: "Occupational therapy practitioners shall use procedures that conform to the standards of practice and other appropriate AOTA documents relevant to practice." The Guidelines to the Occupational Therapy Code of Ethics (1998b) specifically address competence in Standard 4. This companion document to the Code of Ethics indicates that individuals are expected to work within their areas of competence and to pursue opportunities to increase their level of knowledge and skill. In doing so, individuals are expected to engage in appropriate study and to train under supervision before incorporating new interventions into practice. One must consider whether quickly reading an instruction manual was "engaging in appropriate study."

What Actions May Be Taken and What Are the Possible Consequences?

Mr. Murphy could have followed the ethical precepts of Principle 2 of the AOTA Code of Ethics: nonmaleficence, which is avoiding harm. If he had followed this principle, he would have asked for help with Ms. Sonderheim's treatment, or he could have deferred the treatment to another day.

The case does not say whether Mr. Murphy attempted to provide Ms. Sonderheim with an informed choice. Choices are based on informed consent, where one can consent or refuse to take an action. Within the context of health care, recipients of service may consent to treatment after a discussion of possible risks and benefits. The discussion should be in language understandable to all concerned, so that the consent is truly "informed." By involving the client, Mr. Murphy could have elicited a voluntary agreement from Ms. Sonderheim to come back another day or to have another practitioner see her or assist with the treatment. The client could also have refused the treatment. Occupational therapy practitioners must respect the rights of service recipients to act as autonomous individuals. Principle 3.C reads: "the occupational therapy practitioner shall obtain informed consent" and 3.D mention, respecting the right of potential recipients of service to refuse treatment.

In the scenario, the question of honesty should be considered. The Guidelines to the Occupational Therapy Code of Ethics (1998b) note that practitioners should be honest with themselves and know their strengths and limitations. Mr. Murphy should have provided Ms. Sonderheim with several options for her to consider. Telling the truth about one's level of competence and experience may be awkward and risk-laden, but a practitioner is bound to follow the ethics principles concerned with informed consent, veracity, and fidelity. Veracity or truth telling includes informing clients of the practitioner's credentials and skills. The therapeutic relationship is predicated on the assumption that practitioners will act in the best interests of clients (i.e., with fidelity) and that practitioners have the necessary skills and knowledge to help clients improve their level of functioning. In Mr. Murphy's case, what are the consequences, if any, of not telling the truth? Was Mr. Murphy's failure to tell Ms. Sonderheim the level of his expertise a lie by omission.

Nevertheless, Mr. Murphy does have the right to safeguard his own interests and to contact his malpractice carrier to gain a fuller understanding of any liability, rights, and responsibilities. Contacting his malpractice insurer does not indicate liability, guilt, or innocence. Rather, it is something that should be done when facts are fresh in one's mind and a clear recitation of the facts can be given. Mr. Murphy may also contact AOTA's ethics office (if he is a member of AOTA), the NBCOT Disciplinary Action Committee, or the state occupational therapy licensing board to try to clarify his situation. He should recognize that in so doing, however, there is a risk that he may be exposing himself to action by any or all of these entities.

Study Questions

1. What is considered appropriate use of physical agent modalities in occupational therapy?

2. What dictates a profession's domain of practice and scope of practice?

3. Under which circumstances may a practitioner decide not to use a modality that appears to be in the best interests of the client?

4. In the absence of an employing physician and with an ambiguous medical situation, who should the practitioner rely on for supervision and guidance?

5. Under what circumstances is the selection of a therapeutic modality a legal, ethical, or moral dilemma? Which standards outweigh others?

6. How difficult is it to inform a client regarding a practitioner's level of competence? Is failure to do so lying by omission?

Chapter 7

Omnibus Budget Reconciliation Act

CASE: Restraints in the Nursing Home

with commentaries by **Scott Trudeau, MS, OTR,** *and* **Penny Kyler, MA, OTR, FAOTA**

Key Terms

Minimum Data Set (MDS)
Omnibus Budget Reconciliation
   Act

Physical restraint
Resident Assessment
   Instrument (RAI)

CASE: Restraints in the Nursing Home

Ronald Brown's father recently sustained a head injury in a car accident, and the Browns have been caring for him in their home for several months. This arrangement is causing some difficulty because one of the children has had to move out of her bedroom to make room for Mr. Brown. In addition, the Browns are finding their father's behavior disruptive to their routine.

The family felt able to cope with the problems until Mr. Brown began engaging in unsafe activities, such as turning on the stove and forgetting about it, wandering around the house during the night, and even leaving the house during the day and getting lost. On one occasion they found Mr. Brown on the floor next to his bed. The Browns felt obliged to look into nursing home placement, but they were horrified to find that an otherwise pleasant nursing home near them stated that restraint would have to be used some of the time to care for Mr. Brown. The nursing home administrator explained that there were too many residents for the staff to provide individual supervision all the time and that occasionally they had to physically restrain those residents that the staff believed were harmful to themselves or others.

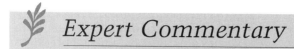

Expert Commentary

By Scott Trudeau, MS, OTR

Introduction

Accepting the fact that a loved one requires admission to a long-term facility is profoundly difficult for families. Much guilt and angst is often experienced, especially when family members make promises to do everything possible to avoid nursing home placement. Perhaps this avoidance is rooted in the fact that care provision in nursing home units in the United States has been in a state of upheaval in the last 15 years. Many factors have contributed to this turmoil, including changes in reimbursement structures, decreases in inpatient lengths of stay, and increasing emphasis on patients' rights and autonomy, to name a few. With the advent of managed care and an increased emphasis on consumerism in health care, further reform to the healthcare delivery system in the United States was inevitable. Nursing home care has not been immune to this reform.

When considering the concerns in the case, it seems necessary to break the issues down. First, there is a need to understand the specifics of the Nursing Home Reform Act (NHRA) and its mandates. Second, one must explore the therapeutic benefits versus the risks of restraint used as an intervention. Finally, some of the recent literature concerning alternative methods of intervention will be considered.

Regulations Governing Nursing Home Care

Historical Perspective

Historically, nursing home oversight had been the purview of each individual state before passage of federal Medicare and Medicaid legislation in 1965. At that time, quality of care varied widely from one state to the next, and regulatory enforcement was inconsistent. In an effort to improve equity and quality of care, federal regulations for skilled nursing facilities (SNFs) were issued in 1974. Despite this regulation, concern persisted into the 1980s regarding the poor quality of nursing home care.

After several highly publicized cases of substandard nursing home care in the 1970s and early 1980s, and the genesis of consumer advocacy groups such as the National Coalition for Nursing Home Reform, pressure mounted for the Health Care Financing Administration (HCFA, now the Centers for Medicare and Medicaid Services [CMS]) to take action. Within this context, in 1983 Congress requested that the Institutes of Medicine (IOM) generate recommendations to improve the quality of nursing home care throughout the United States.

The IOM report, published in 1986 and titled *Improving the Quality of Nursing Home Care*, described many examples of unacceptable care provision in the nursing home industry. In addition, the report highlighted a series of recommendations, which at the request of Congress served as the basis for nursing home regulatory change (Elon & Pawlson, 1992). These recommendations emphasized a significant shift from prior regulatory processes, which focused on documented compliance, to the present focus on outcomes of care and quality indicators.

OBRA 1987

In 1987 the Omnibus Budget Reconciliation Act (OBRA) included legislation addressing quality-of-care issues in nursing homes (Box 7-1). Much of the change in long-term care service delivery can be directly linked to the implementation of the NHRA in 1990, an amendment within OBRA of 1987 (HCFA, 1989). The NHRA sets forth multiple standards to improve the quality of care, the centerpoint being the manner in which resident assessment is completed.

Box 7-1 **By the Law**

The Omnibus Budget Reconciliation Act (OBRA) is legislation addressing quality-of-care issues in nursing homes.

Box 7-2 **Summary**

OBRA legislation includes regulations and standards as well as interpretive guidelines to demonstrate implementation.

It is important to note that the OBRA (1987) legislation has two components that influence care provision in an SNF. First, regulations and standards are defined within the legislation. In addition, interpretive guidelines can be used to see how the regulations should be implemented (Box 7-2). The interpretive guidelines are used by surveyors when determining a facility's compliance with this legislation. This chapter discusses in detail two specific areas of the NHRA that have direct applications to the described case.

Resident Assessment Instrument: Minimum Data Set

The regulations state that a facility must initially and periodically conduct a comprehensive assessment of each resident's functional capacity. Recognizing that to plan and deliver quality outcomes of care, the interdisciplinary team must first properly and comprehensively assess the individual needs of each resident using the **Resident Assessment Instrument (RAI)**. The regulation dictates that this assessment process include the resident's:

- ▶ Medical history
- ▶ Current medical status
- ▶ Functional status
- ▶ Sensory and physical impairments
- ▶ Nutritional status and requirements
- ▶ Special treatments and procedures
- ▶ Psychosocial status
- ▶ Discharge potential
- ▶ Dental condition
- ▶ Activities potential
- ▶ Rehabilitation potential
- ▶ Cognitive status
- ▶ Drug therapy

Comprehensive assessment must occur within 14 days of admission and must be repeated annually or when a significant change in functional status of the resident occurs.

To ensure compliance with this regulation, the **Minimum Data Set (MDS)** assessment protocol, developed via contract from the HCFA, is used. The MDS defines an interdisciplinary evaluative process that is completed within defined timelines. Throughout the MDS process, a variety of issues may be identified that will initiate further assessment. A total of 18 Resident Assessment Protocols (RAPs) can be triggered within the MDS process (Table 7-1). When an area is triggered, in-depth assessment is used to determine the appropriate interventions for the resident and response from the treatment team.

As a result of these OBRA mandates and the interpretive guidelines, the Brown family should be assured that their loved one will have a comprehensive evaluation of his individual needs upon admission to a long-term care facility. The evaluative process directly considers risk for falls, indications for **physical restraints,** and rehabilitation potential, all of which seem to be concerns expressed in this case (Box 7-3). At this stage, occupational therapy intervention is initiated. As a key member of the interdisciplinary team, the occupational therapy practitioner contributes much to the assessment of the resident's functional status. The assessment becomes the foundation for a treatment plan specifically designed to address the client's individual needs.

Box 7-3 *Summary*

The evaluative process directly considers risk for falls, indications for physical restraints, and rehabilitation potential.

Physical Restraint Regulations

Few areas of the NHRA are as controversial as the regulations directly pertaining to the use of restraint in nursing home populations. OBRA clearly states that residents have a right to be free of physical restraints imposed for purposes of discipline or convenience and not required to

Table 7–1
Resident Assessment Protocols

1.	Delirium
2.	Cognitive loss/dementia
3.	Visual function
4.	Communication
5.	Activities of daily living (ADL) function/rehabilitative potential
6.	Urinary incontinence and indwelling catheter
7.	Psychosocial well-being
8.	Mood state
9.	Behavioral problems
10.	Activities
11.	Falls
12.	Nutritional status
13.	Feeding tubes
14.	Dehydration/fluid maintenance
15.	Dental care
16.	Pressure ulcer
17.	Antipsychotic drug use
18.	Physical restraints

treat a specific medical symptom (Tag number F203/Regulation number 483.13(a), HCFA, 1989). A physical or mechanical restraint is defined as any device attached or adjacent to one's body that restricts freedom of movement or normal access to one's body (HCFA, 1992). By definition a wide variety of materials could be classified as restraints, including vests, belts, wrist/ankle straps, sheets, bed rails, or geriatric chairs with fixed tray tables. Any time an individual is not able to easily release the device and voluntarily regain freedom of movement, the definition of physical restraint has been met.

Compliance with the OBRA mandates requires that facilities consider and document all less-restrictive alternatives that have been attempted before employing the physical restraint. Decisions regarding the necessity of restraint use must be directly based on the RAI-MDS process described previously. Through this process the team determines the indications for restraints and outlines the less-restrictive alternatives that may be appropriate to consider.

Patterns of Restraint Use

Because regulation of nursing home practices was inconsistent, there was likewise inconsistent data available to reliably report trends in restraint use. Evans and Strumpf (1989) conducted one of the first comprehensive literature reviews to elucidate issues of restraint use in the elderly. Although these authors note that restraint use was relatively commonplace in long-term care settings, reporting prevalence ranging from 25 to 84.6 percent, literature or evidence to support such widespread use of restraints was scarce. It became clear in this literature review that certain resident attributes can be predictive of restraint use. The three risk factors predictive of restraint use in nursing homes most commonly cited in the early literature include age, cognitive impairment, and behavioral symptoms (Box 7-4). Based on this pre-OBRA literature, Mr. Brown could clearly be considered at risk of being physically restrained in most nursing homes in the mid-1980s.

Box 7-4 Summary

Three risk factors predictive of restraint use in nursing homes include age, cognitive impairment, and behavioral symptoms.

Rationale for Restraint Use

The underlying principle referred to in the literature to justify the use of restraint is protection: to protect the patient from incurring an injury from a fall, from harming him or herself or someone else, from interfering with medical intervention such as a feeding tube, and so on. Although many clinicians believe that the aim of protection justifies the intervention from a moral standpoint, evidence often suggests that the opposite is true. For instance, Tinetti, Liu, Maratolli, and Ginter (1991) reported that the notion that restraints would decrease falls or fall-related injuries was unfounded. Persons at high risk for falls actually fell more often when restraints were used.

Restraint-Reduction Initiatives

The myths associated with restraint use must be dispelled through both evidence and education. Effective programs for restraint reduction can be used to help in this effort. In addition, for restraint-reduction efforts to be successful, realistic and practical alternatives must be available for managing the risks and behaviors traditionally addressed with a physical restraint intervention. Unfortunately, the expectation voiced by the Browns that staff coverage be increased to allow for one-to-one supervision is often not practical, nor has it been proven to be optimally effective in reducing injuries (Janelli, Kanski, & Neary, 1994).

Deleterious Effects of Physical Restraint

With the regulatory scrutiny that is being focused on nursing homes, research describing the harmful effects of restraint use has increased. Restricting a person's mobility alone results in a wide range of negative physical and psychological consequences for the person being restrained (Table 7-2). Risk-benefit analysis makes it profoundly difficult to rationalize the use of restraints. As the lack of evidence to support the benefits of restraints becomes apparent, and with the knowledge that their use has been associated with multiple forms of death, can this intervention in a care environment be justified? Education programs must confront these realities so that care providers and families such as the Browns can be empowered to weigh the risks and benefits effectively (Dunbar, Neufeld, White, & Libow, 1996).

Clinical Decision Making

Miles and Myers (1994) outline a process for clinical decision making regarding restraint use. Their model highlights two points that are consistent with many of the NHRA regulations and seems useful to consider in the Brown case. First, the care plan must be individualized, which requires comprehensive evaluation of the situation by the interdisciplinary team to determine how restraint use will benefit the elderly person.

The next step Miles and Myers propose involves informed consent. There are three components to consent, including (1) the symptom or

Table 7–2
Potential for Harm from Restraint Use

Psychological Effects	Functional Impacts	Injuries
Stress	Immobility	Ligature strangulation
Fear	Deconditioning	Asphyxiation
Humiliation	Incontinence	Nerve injuries
Agitation	Skin breakdown	Fall trauma
Combativeness	Increased infections	Intestinal infarction
Demoralization	Bone demineralization	Skin abrasions
Anger	Joint contractures	Contusions
Learned dependence	Edema	
	Decreased circulation	
	Decreased appetite	
	Constipation	

Box 7-5 *Summary*

Three components of consent include the symptom or need for the intervention, the benefits of the restraint, and the potential for adverse effects of the restraint.

need for the intervention, (2) the benefits of the restraint and how the resident's well-being will be enhanced, and (3) the potential for adverse effects of the restraint (Box 7-5). Because this chapter noted earlier that the prevalence of restraint use increases proportionately with cognitive impairment, the consent process often includes the need for proxy decision making and education regarding risks and benefits of the intervention. The treatment team must ensure that the Brown family is knowledgeable for them to advocate for the best care for their loved one.

Alternatives to Restraint

The primary resource for developing alternatives to restraints in an institution again relates to the interdisciplinary assessment of each individual. The potential for alternatives is as vast as the number of reasons they might be needed and the individuals who might employ them. To develop the most effective alternatives, the interdisciplinary team members must blend their expertise to identify the core problems and then creatively resolve these issues. Table 7-3 may be useful to highlight some examples of alternatives to restraint use.

Conclusion

The Brown case highlights all of the issues presented in this chapter. The occupational therapist has an opportunity to participate with the treatment team in evaluating Mr. Brown and educating the staff and family, to dispel myths about restraint use. The occupational therapy practitioner has a key role to play in developing creative solutions for the behavioral problems that may arise for Mr. Brown. Recommendations for environmental adaptations and development of an adequate routine of daily occupations will be important if Mr. Brown is to be cared for without resorting to the use of restraints.

The occupational therapist must work closely with physical therapists to develop interventions aimed at promoting functional mobility. Assessing and developing improved balance and strength, and finding safe transfer techniques to maximize Mr. Brown's physical abilities, will be essential. Once an assessment of the need for skilled interventions is complete, the occupational therapist must communicate with the team (especially the direct care staff) to establish strategies to ensure that Mr. Brown maintains progress. The Brown family will also benefit from the expertise of the occupational therapy practitioner by receiving education regarding the functional status of their loved one and by learning strategies to ensure his safety while avoiding restraint.

Table 7–3
Examples of Restraint Alternatives

Environmental Alterations	Patient Care Approaches	Activity Promotion
Door alarms	Validation	ADL involvement
Seating alarms	Anticipation of needs	Structured social opportunity
Camouflaged exits	Individualized care plan	Routine and structure
Safe wandering paths	Toileting schedules	Fitness involvement
Adequate lighting	Ambulation schedules	Walking
Regulated temperature	Avoid unnecessary conflicts	Music
Anti-tip wheelchairs	Medication management	Rehabilitation when indicated
High-low beds		
Customized seating		

How can occupational therapy practitioners help nursing home residents? Accurate diagnosis of the nursing home resident is important; however, functional status is also important. With the advent of OBRA, the focus has shifted from "doing for" to "working with" residents. Occupational therapy practitioners are qualified to train staff to help enhance residents' autonomy.

The clinician's focus on the residents' functional status—both physical and mental—can have a positive effect on both residents and staff. When staff members are trained as enablers rather than doers, their jobs are less burdensome. To bring about this change, occupational therapy practitioners can lead staff training sessions with a focus on environmental adaptation and can teach functional activities to promote independence. They can also help nursing home staff members to establish and implement an intervention plan for the elderly resident that respects his or her autonomy.

🌿 *Ethical Commentary*

By Penny Kyler, MA, OTR, FAOTA

This case of restraints in the nursing home raises one of the most difficult issues that some adult children have to face: whether to put their parent into a nursing home. Fears of death, disability, the aging process, and diminishing finances are just a sample of the issues confronting them. These issues may also be experienced by therapists in their personal lives and may color their professional judgment and actions, both professionally when they are working with elderly clients and personally when they are faced with their own dilemma such as the one presented in this case.

The intent of the various federal regulations regarding nursing homes (OBRA and HCFA/CMS) is to improve the quality of care for those in nursing homes. The Browns may not feel completely comfortable with their choice, but they should feel better that their decision to place Mr. Brown in a nursing home is governed by standards that dictate quality of care. Notification upfront that this particular nursing home does use physical restraints provides information and makes the Browns informed consumers. Remember that Mr. Brown's freedom would not be unduly restricted as long as he was acting in a safe manner. Also, he would be in an environment where his movements could be monitored and where staff could help ensure his safety. The Brown family may wish to interview other staff members in the nursing home and to visit several times before admitting their father to see if resident autonomy and family collaboration with treatment were truly honored.

Who Are the Players?

The Browns, their children, their father, the nursing home staff, other nursing home residents, the nursing home administrator, and the physicians are the players. Are there any others?

What Other Information Is Needed?

What is Mr. Brown's level of functional independence? What are his favorite daily occupations, and will he be able to participate in any of them in the nursing home? What type of environmental assessment has been done in the home? What home health and social services are available? What social supports are available for Ronald Brown and his family? What is the physician's prognosis for Mr. Brown? How many nursing homes have the younger Browns visited? Are there financial considerations? What other options are available to the Browns if they decide against the nursing home? What level of care does Mr. Brown need?

What Actions May Be Taken and What Are the Possible Consequences?

The younger Browns are facing a dilemma because they have to make a decision with no obvious best answer. Everyone makes decisions that touch other people's lives. These decisions often leave people wondering whether they are doing the right thing. Questions arise such as: "Is this decision meeting the needs of all the people involved?" Some people feel comfortable only if all questions are decided by persons in positions of authority, who they believe have the right answer. Rightness and wrongness play very strong roles in human decision making.

In deciding this case, the Browns should ask: What are the facts for Mr. Brown, for themselves, for their children, and for the nursing home administration and staff? No one has the exact same set of values and beliefs, so that facts take on as many colors and shapes as there are people looking at the situation. The Browns should view all the facts given to them as *interpreted* facts. Facts have meaning based on individual histories and the context in which the fact is given. Each person's history influences how he or she interprets things. In this case, the facts are influenced by the connectedness of the players—father to son, husband to wife, father and mother to children, grandfather to granddaughter, and so on—as well as the events in the home that led up to the inquiry about nursing home placement.

Facts are interpreted differently. The stronger people feel about something, the more important it is to listen to what others have to say. People who disagree are not always wrong, and other people may feel equally as strongly about their interpretation of the facts. Individuals must try to accept the fallibility of their moral choices because choices are rarely either totally right or totally wrong. People can evaluate how much physical and emotional energy they wish to put into making a decision about a set of facts because they evaluate facts in light of how important they are to them personally.

In looking at the facts surrounding the Brown case, Ronald Brown must decide if the facts warrant nursing home placement for his father. He can ask: Does the action (putting his father in a nursing home) fit the situation (the problems at home)? Or are there other alternatives? What is the least restrictive and best environment for his father? Had Mr. Brown junior had prior discussions with his father before his father's brain injury? Does he know or at least have a good idea about what his father's wishes would be in this type of situation?

As part of his fact finding, Ronald Brown should be able to access a report of the chosen nursing home to see staffing patterns, safety violations, and the level of care provided. Gathering all the facts will help him make a better decision.

Regarding occupational therapy interventions, if Mr. Brown becomes a resident of the nursing home, Mr. Trudeau's discussion of occupational therapy nicely covers potential benefits from those services. Readers may wish to consider Principle 1 of the Occupational Therapy Code of Ethics, which indicates that practitioners collaborate with recipients of service throughout the intervention process. Mr. Brown senior is the primary recipient of service.

Study Questions

1. Regulations state that a facility must initially and periodically conduct a comprehensive assessment of each resident's functional capacity. What areas are addressed in the assessment?

2. Compliance with the OBRA mandates requires that facilities consider and document all less-restrictive alternatives that have been attempted before employing the physical restraint. How is physical restraint defined?

3. What are the three risk factors predictive of restraint use in nursing homes most commonly cited in the early literature?

4. What are the therapeutic benefits versus risks of restraint use as an intervention?

5. What are the three components of consent if the use of restraints is indicated?

6. What alternatives exist to the use of restraints?

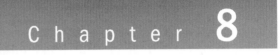

Chapter 8

Confidentiality in Groups: Ethical Dilemmas and Possible Resolutions

CASE: **Caregiver Support Group**

with commentaries by **Nina D. Fieldsteel, PhD,**
and **Penny Kyler, MA, OTR, FAOTA**

Key Terms

Agreement of confidentiality   Ethics
Ethical dilemmas   Group contact

CASE: Caregiver Support Group

A caregiver support group has been running for 8 weeks. The purpose of the group is to provide education and support to technical-level personnel providing care for elders with Alzheimer's disease. An occupational therapist coleads the group with a psychologist.

One of the group members, an occupational therapy aide, was recently divorced from an occupational therapist who is coincidentally a supervisor to some of the other group members. In the hospital cafeteria, the psychologist overhears this group member's ex-wife talking with another group member about the aide's abusiveness during their marriage. At the group's next meeting, the aide opens the group sobbing. He explains that his ex-wife has succeeded in gaining full custody of their child. Deeply distressed, he is having difficulty caring for his patients. He exclaims, "She is a lying bitch, and now I have lost my child." What are the concerns related to confidentiality in this group?

What issues are raised concerning confidentiality in therapy groups and support groups? What are the legal and ethical considerations for the members, group leaders, agency, and associated professionals?

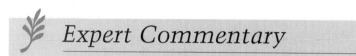

Expert Commentary

By Nina D. Fieldsteel, PhD

Introduction

The ethical dilemmas posed in this vignette are many. The first set of dilemmas relate to the structure of the group, its definition, setting, and origin, and the problems of dual, even multiple relationships among and between group members and leaders. The second set of dilemmas relates to the reported incident in the cafeteria. They involve the role of the leader, the role of a supervisor, and other boundary issues. The last set of dilemmas is posed by the events within the group. They concern the need for choices when faced with both clinical and ethical issues.

The many dilemmas in this clinical vignette involve different aspects of confidentiality, group boundaries, and dual relationships. Ethical dilemmas are those situations in which there are no clear definitions of right or wrong (Box 8-1). The clinician has to be guided by those principles of ethical behavior that are commonly held by mental health professionals.

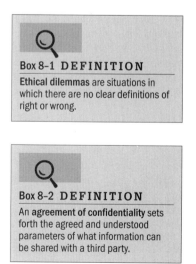

Box 8-1 DEFINITION

Ethical dilemmas are situations in which there are no clear definitions of right or wrong.

Box 8-2 DEFINITION

An agreement of confidentiality sets forth the agreed and understood parameters of what information can be shared with a third party.

Among the basic principles are: (1) to do no harm, (2) to value the individual and to respect individual differences, and (3) to maintain and defend the confidentiality of the exchanges between the patient (client or group member) and the therapist (counselor or group leader) (Box 8-2). Confidentiality is considered essential to any therapeutic effort.

Ethics is a code of behavior (Box 8-3). It deals with actions—with what ought to be. Behavior is evaluated in relation to moral principles and values. These moral principles have been developed both by the individual and by society over time and from an understanding of the intentions and consequences of those actions.

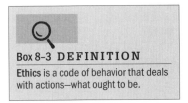

Box 8-3 DEFINITION

Ethics is a code of behavior that deals with actions—what ought to be.

It is necessary to be aware of the fact that sometimes legal definitions of acceptable behavior may differ from ethical principles. There are times when behavior that is considered ethically important is not legally protected. In each instance, commonly held guidelines and principles of group practice, the role of the leader, and the implied obligations of the group members to one another and to the group must be considered. The overriding concern of the group leader is for the needs of the group members and for what is required for them to have a growth-enhancing experience.

Dilemmas Related to the Structure of the Group

This group consists of individuals working within the same institution, possibly within the same unit. Several questions have to be answered because they determine the structure of the group and shape the ethical parameters.

Who set up this group: the institution, the leaders, or did the members indicate the need for such a group? Are the group leaders also employees of the same institution or are they independent professionals who were brought in to lead the group? What are their obligations to the institution? Are the usual limits of confidentiality agreed upon by the group leaders and their institutional employers? Is membership in the group voluntary or prescribed? What obligations do the group leaders have to the institution? What prior or continuing relationships do they have with some or all of the group members?

In setting up a group within an institution for staff education, development, and support, these questions have to be answered before the group members, the leaders, and the institution can expect a successful result from such an undertaking. In the current group literature, the term *contract* is frequently used to describe the agreed upon and fully understood parameters of the group (Rutan & Stone, 1984) (Box 8-4). The parameters are the composition of the membership, the role of the leaders

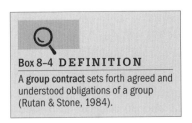

Box 8-4 DEFINITION

A **group contract** sets forth agreed and understood obligations of a group (Rutan & Stone, 1984).

and their obligations to both the group members and the institution, and the obligations of the members to the group, to one another and to the leaders. These contracts are often just verbal agreements. At present, the 2000 Health Insurance Portability and Accountability Act (HIPAA) laws (APA, 2002) require a written contract. Whether written or verbal, the ethical principle behind such a contract is that all of the parties to the contract are clear about the obligations and limits of the shared undertaking.

Clearly there is a vast difference between a group that is set up by the institution as part of staff training and support, with leaders who have no reporting or supervisory function, and in which the group membership is voluntary, and one that is required by the employer and is understood by both members and leaders as serving to evaluate performance and may even determine continued employment. The group structure has to be clearly defined and its goals agreed upon by the group members for it to function successfully. The relationship of the group leaders to the institutional setting has to be clarified as a necessary condition for developing trust and ensuring confidentiality in the group. For any group working together to try to understand their relationship within the workplace and with one another, the integrity of the group and the trust in the boundaries of the group's agreement about confidentiality are essential. Trust can only be built up over time by repeated incidents and actions that confirm the group leaders' commitment to maintaining confidentiality.

The assumption of and the protection of confidentiality between the individual and the psychologist, social worker, or psychiatrist has long been established. The recent Supreme Court ruling (*Jaffee* v. *Redmond*, 1996) extended that protection to include not only licensed professionals but also others who are clearly serving in the position of counselor or in a helping role. The legal limitations of confidentially differ in each state. Regulations established under state law, such as the Tarasoff decision, and laws about reporting child abuse, sexual and spousal abuse, and HIV/AIDS all may vary by state. It is therefore necessary to be aware of the laws in your particular state.

There is an even more important legal limitation to confidentiality relating to work in groups. Legally defined, *confidentiality* is limited to the individual patient and the therapist. It is not considered protected when information is shared in the presence of a third person. Under this definition, information shared in couples, family, or group therapy is not protected. In groups, it becomes the task of the leader to define clearly for the group the rules of confidentiality that will be observed in the group. Although not legally binding, the rules of confidentiality are assumed to be ethically and morally binding for all group members and for the leader.

It becomes the task of the group leader to be alert to any breaks in this agreement. For example, a member may say something like, "I told my wife about your problems and she was so sympathetic." Although this action was not malicious in intent, it still has to be discussed as a violation of the group agreement of confidentiality. This attention to breaks in confidentiality, even when "innocent," reinforces the importance of confidentiality to the whole group. In a well-functioning group, group members will eventually be alert to such breaks and attend to them. The rule that "what is talked about in the group stays in the group" is reinforced and becomes central to the group members' sense of safety and trust.

In this group, because members work in the same place, the usual boundary definitions cannot apply. Members see one another outside of the group and have multiple relationships in the workplace. They may even have developed social relationships outside of work in their previous time together before starting group. These relationships have to be acknowledged and shared with the group. The leaders have to be sensitive to how these relationships may affect group interactions.

It is helpful if there are several groups being formed at the same time, that close friends or supervisors and supervisees be separated. If it is not possible, then it is important to closely observe the rule stated previously of keeping group material within the group. The corollary principle that "whenever a group matter is discussed outside the group, it is to be brought back into the group" serves to maintain the group boundaries. Of necessity, the definition of what is group material is periodically reconsidered and redefined.

Box 8-5 *Summary*

The ethical task is to examine issues of confidentiality, group boundaries, and dual relationships.

The possibilities of dual relationships with the leader or leaders are also an important issue in workplace-based groups. Here too the ethical task is to define and clarify the boundaries of the relationship of the leader(s) to the members and to the institution (Box 8-5).

The Dilemmas Presented by the Incident in the Cafeteria

The exchange in the cafeteria, as described in the reported vignette, presented many ethical dilemmas. Do the leaders wait for the group member to report the event to the group? Does she then have the opportunity to explore within the group what it felt like to be given this information about a fellow group member? Does the leader take the initiative and report to the group what he or she overheard? Does this provide the opportunity to help group members learn ways to maintain the group's boundaries?

In this group session, as reported, neither the group member nor the leader had a chance to talk about the incident. The spontaneous, tearful account of his wife's behavior by the distressed husband precluded any other discussion. It reaffirms the wisdom of the suggestion that breaks in confidentiality or other group rules take precedence in group discussion. This incident also illustrates the fact that it is not always possible to predict or control what will happen in a group. In a new group, such as this one, dealing with these issues immediately, as they arise, can emphasize how important it is to resolve these issues for the group to function well and reaffirms the leaders' serious intention to preserve the group's boundaries. Because this did not occur and the husband began with his distress, the leaders' clinical judgment and skill will have to be relied on in deciding when to introduce the information that one leader overheard and that a group member was given unsolicited. Other implications of this event will be discussed in the next section on dilemmas.

One of the important things the leader can model for the group, in bringing up the incident at the beginning of the group, is how to stop such unsolicited exchanges. The group member might ask, "What could I do? She began talking and I couldn't stop her." Letting the group members deal with this question can be useful for all of them because such an incident is likely to happen in groups within a close work community.

Ethical Dilemmas Created by the Events in the Group

Some of the ethical dilemmas presented by the distressing information that the husband shared would be determined by how the group and the leaders might have responded to his material. It would be useful to know the distribution of men and women in the group. Were the two leaders men, women, or a man and a woman?

The introduction of the information about the cafeteria incident adds to the complicated situation. How will it affect the husband's feeling of trust in the group? The leaders' skill and sensitivity will be needed to help the group member share with the group what she had been told by the ex-wife. The situation will have to be timed so that the husband does not feel further diminished and betrayed by the group. Will his ex-wife become an intrusive presence in the group, a threat not only to him and his relationship with his child but also an interference with his work in the group?

In this attempt to deal with an ethical issue, clinical skills and the necessity to protect a vulnerable group member are important factors in determining what is "right." The timing is essential because the even more important ethical guideline "do no harm" takes precedence here.

The leaders are concerned not only with what is ethically correct, but also with what will be helpful to the group member. When is it appropriate to introduce this necessary but difficult new information to the group member? Here it would be important for the leaders to know the group members, their strengths, and their vulnerabilities. It would also be important to know how the leaders saw the members' relationships within the group. Were they mutually supportive and friendly? Were subgroups developing in the group? Was aggression and competitiveness being enacted in the group? The resolution of these dilemmas depends on a multiplicity of factors.

Summary 🌿

The various ethical dilemmas have been noted and hopefully clarified. There are no simple solutions. The actions that were suggested are, at best, only suggestions. Any attempt to resolve such dilemmas is always strengthened by adequate information about the group and its members.

In a new group, the emphasis has to be on defining what is necessary to allow the group to develop trust and good working relationships. A clear definition of the group's goals, the boundaries that define the group, and the importance of maintaining confidentiality take precedence.

If practitioners try to be guided by the principles of respect and caring, valuing individual differences, and the importance of confidentiality in developing trust, they are most likely to remain within the boundaries of ethical behavior. Wallerstein (1976) quotes a statement from Harris Chaiklin: "We are only ethical when we are constantly worrying about what is right; *that is the burden of being a professional*" (p. 372). The discussion of this clinical vignette and its problems is evidence that even in what seems like a simple situation, there is a lot to worry about. There may be no easy solutions; however, a discussion of ethical dilemmas helps heighten practitioners' awareness of both ethical and clinical issues.

🌿 *Ethical Commentary*

By Penny Kyler, MA, OTR, FAOTA

Who Are the Players?

In this scenario the players include the members of the support group, the occupational therapist and psychologist coleaders, the occupational therapy aide, the occupational therapist ex-wife of the aide, and the group member in whom she confided. Are there any others?

What Other Information is Needed?

The information stated and the issues fleshed out by Dr. Fieldsteel, such as the role of the supervisor and boundary awareness, are inclusive; however, one should also consider other avenues for exploration. As an example, could the occupational therapy aide be referred to an employee assistance program? Could the couple be placed in different parts of the facility? Do the occupational therapy ex-wife and all group members have an understanding of ethics and confidentiality? Has any of the domestic unrest affected patient treatment and care? Have any others in the occupational therapy department been affected by the disagreement? Were the boundaries of the group clearly defined? Do other issues affect this scenario?

What Actions May Be Taken, and What Are the Possible Consequences?

The preamble to the Occupational Therapy Code of Ethics (2000a) clearly indicates that the Code does apply to personnel, including staff such as aides, orderlies, and clerical staff. The question is whether personal issues that do not affect patient care are covered within the context of the Code. This outburst by the occupational therapy aide was personal in nature and was not done in front of patients, nor was it done within the time frame and context of a therapeutic group (this is a support group). Should that incident be considered a breach of occupational therapy ethics? The aide and his ex-wife work as colleagues in the same facility and probably have both work and social relations in common with other group members. It is unknown whether the topics of divorce, abusive behavior, child custody, and so on have come up in the group. Thus it is also unknown whether these concerns are part of what the aide should be legitimately discussing in the group and which would therefore be covered by group confidentiality.

The larger or more general issue is one of confidentiality on the part of the aide's ex-wife—an occupational therapist who supervises some of the group members. Was her discussion with a group member in the cafeteria a breach of confidentiality? Many of us know of individuals who have had "bad days" and have shared their personal concerns with coworkers. The generally accepted boundaries of privacy have also expanded as individuals use cellular phones in public to discuss what only a few years ago would be considered private and personal matters.

Generally, students in health professions are taught the importance of confidentiality and boundaries. Those who speak openly of patients in public areas, such as a facility cafeteria, are admonished, but a practitioner who shares personal information is usually ignored. Of course, personal conversation is generally not a breach of professional confidentiality; however, it might be considered so in this scenario because the therapist supervises some of her ex-husband's colleagues. The concern in this scenario might be that if the occupational therapist ex-wife does not recognize her comments as a breach of personal ethics, would she recognize them as a breach in professional ethics? In the AOTA's code of professional ethics, Principle 7 indicates that practitioners should treat their colleagues with fairness, discretion, and integrity, and Principle 7.A says practitioners should safeguard confidential information. Speaking openly of personal issues to one's supervisee in a public area shows not only a lack of tact and discretion but is also a breach of the Code of Ethics concerning safeguarding confidential information and treating a colleague with fairness and integrity.

Conclusion

This scenario can be seen from the viewpoints of a variety of ethics theories. One such theory is ethical subjectivism, in which right and wrong are viewed as relative based on the attitudes of each person (Percesepe, 1995). Some philosophers disagree with this perspective because if people took this view about everything, they would never have to be responsible for their actions and would in essence be infallible. Another lens through which to view the scenario is that of social contract ethics. Social contract ethics takes the position that people must live in this society together and that the actions of one person affect others. Because everyone must live together, there must be rules regarding how to do so successfully. If there were no rules and general agreements, living conditions would likely dissolve into chaos (Percesepe, 1995).

No matter how one looks at this scenario, no action wrapped within a personal problem is simple on a conceptual basis. Individuals will each view the same scenario in different ways; questions such as what is he really doing and why, or what is she really doing and why may be answered in a multitude of ways. Their actions may be as a result of their history or they may be current spontaneity. The scenario must be put in the context of occupational therapy ethics and more specifically in the place where professional ethics intersect with personal ethics in the context of confidentiality and group process, as discussed by Dr. Fieldsteel. In this scenario, issues related to confidentiality and group process need to be constantly in the forefront of the leaders' minds because the complexity of personal and professional ethics among these group members and their supervisors may at some point cross over to patient care.

Study Questions

1. How are aspects of confidentiality, group boundaries, and dual relationships related to ethical behavior on the part of the group leader and members?

2. In what ways might the legal definitions of confidentiality differ from ethical principles or behavior?

3. How can ethical dilemmas related to confidentiality be addressed when considering the structure of a group?

4. How can ethical dilemmas related to confidentiality be addressed when considering the process of a group?

5. What differences exist between educational, support, and therapeutic groups in relation to group contracts around confidentiality? On what basis are these differences determined?

Section **3**

The Manager

In Chapter 9 on rationing of treatment, Daniels and Emanuel illustrate an issue raised in the Ethical Principles section of Chapter 1—that of balancing the competing needs of society. Throughout their discussion, they combine the principles of beneficence (acting in ways that promote the welfare of others) and nonmaleficence (acting in ways that do not cause harm or injury) with the principal of utility (acting in ways that bring about the greatest benefits and the least harm) to establish a guide for satisfying the competing needs of the clients in an elder care facility.

If a practitioner were to follow these principles, he or she would be able to use resources (in this case, time and expertise) to do as much good as possible for elderly clients. Daniels and Emanuel lead us through the considerations needed to achieve such a desirable outcome. Considerations such as the following are raised: deciding which clients are likely to make the most improvement in their functional status; involving as much as possible the payors, clients, and facility administration in decision making; and choosing an action on the basis of a client's individual traits rather than on group profiles or characteristics.

In Chapter 10 on patients' rights, Gutheil implicitly uses the ethical principle of autonomy (rational people have the right to be self-determining) as a framework for his discussion on informed consent. His discussion of the "dangerous patient" brings to light competing duties to the individual patient and the group as a whole. Again, as in Chapter 9, ethical principles of beneficence, nonmaleficence, and utility are considerations in decisions about a patient's right to refuse occupational therapy. This right bears a relationship of risks to others, including staff, family members, and other clients.

Gracey's discussion of informed consent in Chapter 11 presents a practitioner's dual responsibilities when clients are participating in research at the same time as receiving services. The potential for conflict of interests is discussed, stating that practitioners must be clear on their primary responsibility to clients who are receiving intervention under a contract for care. Aspects of the Common Rule are discussed as they relate to the AOTA code of ethics: privacy, confidentiality, and informed consent.

In Schwartzberg's discussion of contracts and referrals to private practice in Chapter 12, the legal concept of what is reasonable (that which is considered customary practice) is emphasized. In consideration of dilemmas imposed by an absence of contracts, practitioners are advised to make explicit agreements.

In his new chapter on the whistleblower (Chapter 13), Gutheil makes clear the valuable role such persons play in health care, explains why they need and deserve special protections against retaliation, and suggests support strategies they might employ. He points out the lonely and difficult road whistleblowers walk while playing their part to see that our most vulnerable citizens are protected from unethical care.

Each of the five chapters in this last section has particular relevance to the occupational therapy manager. Nevertheless, the ethical and legal concepts presented have broad implications for the practitioner, student, and educator.

Chapter 9

Rationing of Treatment

CASE 1: **Triage in an Elder Care Facility**
CASE 2: **Too Many Cases to Handle**
CASE 3: **The Seven-Day Work Week**
with commentary by **Norman Daniels, PhD,**
and **Ezekiel Emanuel, MD, PhD**

Key Terms

Healthcare rationing
Relative benefit

Shotgun approach
Third-party payor

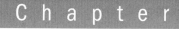

CASE 1: Triage in an Elder Care Facility

Linda works for a large healthcare facility serving elderly people, some of whom are likely to remain in the facility, whereas others are able to return home following rehabilitation. There are 500 residents in the facility and one occupational therapist on the rehabilitation team. Linda has received a "blanket referral" to treat all of the clients who are likely to return home (about 50) and specific referrals to treat those residents who are likely to remain in the facility and who could benefit from rehabilitation services (about 30 clients).

Linda is very interested in using her rehabilitation skills to treat the clients who can return home. They generally make quick gains and are gratifying to work with. Of the other group of clients, however, several could improve their self-care skills considerably, achieving a greater sense of self-worth and independence and relieving the direct care staff of a great deal of work.

Linda cannot possibly treat all of the clients who have been referred to her. She must choose the 30 or so whom she can see. She is not sure what criteria she should use to make her decisions. Whom should she prioritize? The clients who are likely to make the most progress? Those who are likely to return home soonest? Those who could increase their independence quickly in the facility, so that they are less of a burden on staff members and can feel better about themselves? Those about whom the referring physician is most persuasive? Those who are most troublesome to the direct care staff?

CASE 2: Too Many Cases to Handle

Over the past few months, Julio's caseload has been growing. His supervisor expects him to cover a full client load in the hospital and to do home visits as well. Although an additional job has been advertised, there has been little response. Julio suspects that no one wants to work in this inner-city neighborhood clinic. He doesn't mind working at the clinic because he grew up in the neighborhood and he is able to physically care for himself, being large and of strong build; however, he can sympathize with others who might not be as "tough."

One of his home care clients, a known drug dealer on the streets, recently reached a plateau in occupational therapy. Several months earlier he had suffered a stroke from cocaine use. The clinic does not provide treatment unless progress is demonstrated. If Julio documents some minor change while making brief visits, he can continue full treatment sessions when the client starts making progress again. This will allow him to reduce his workload for the moment. As Julio sees it, if therapy is terminated, the client may never get the help he needs in the future. Young female therapists would refuse to go into this neighborhood, especially if they found out the client was a drug dealer. There are no other men in Julio's department, and he believes he has good rapport with the client. In fact, he believes the client may even seek drug counseling if Julio continues his visits.

Is it ethical to document progress in this case? Does the therapist have a moral obligation to the community? By spending less time with the drug dealer client, Julio can be both cost-effective for his department and more effective with his other clients—those in the hospital who are acutely ill. He has discussed the matter with his supervisor, who told him they have no choice but to cover the caseload. What should Julio do, and what is the supervisor's obligation to the client and to the facility?

CASE 3: The Seven-Day Work Week

For the past 6 years Aruzhana Masouk has been the sole occupational therapist on a psychiatric unit in a general hospital. The average length of stay has become shorter and shorter over the years, and it is now about 7 days. There is growing pressure from the unit director and head nurse to have occupational therapy coverage on evenings and weekends. The nursing staff are being asked by the unit director to do activities with clients in the evenings in the occupational therapy room. Aruzhana has resisted allowing the use of occupational therapy supplies by other staff members because she believes these are the therapeutic media of occupational therapy. She has, however, been willing to consult with the nursing staff if they want help in running a recreational program or in planning weekend and evening activities.

The administration will not pay for additional occupational therapy coverage. Aruzhana is a single parent and does not want to give up her precious time with her young daughter to work evenings and weekends. The clients being admitted are more acutely ill than in the past, requiring more individualized attention and evaluations. If Aruzhana runs more groups, rather than individual evaluation and treatment sessions, she risks not meeting the individual needs of the clients. If she works evenings and weekends, her family relationships will suffer. What should she do?

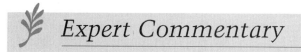

Expert Commentary

By Norman Daniels, PhD, and Ezekiel Emanuel, MD, PhD

[The Expert Commentary for this chapter is an abridged version of an interview, conducted by the editors with Norman Daniels and Ezekiel Emanuel, at the Dana Farber Cancer Research Center in Boston, Massachusetts.]

Sharan Schwartzberg (SS): Let me start by explaining why we wanted to include something in this book on the rationing of treatment (Box 9-1). Members of our profession seem to be more and more interested in ethical questions, and occurrences of unethical behavior are increasing. For example, complaints before our licensure boards and national certification board are growing. So, in the case vignettes for this chapter on rationing, we picked situations that would be difficult for therapists, which they might not be educated to deal with, and in which they would have to make judgments that are not easily made.

> **Box 9-1 Summary**
>
> **Based on finite and limited resources, healthcare rationing is making relative choices about who should receive care.**

Specifically in this chapter, we're concerned with dilemmas in rationing occupational therapy. What are the legal implications resulting from any decisions that are made? What are the professional, client, facility, and societal issues? We would like to see if you could help therapists to think through a dilemma, so that they have a planned basis for action and are able to act more judiciously in the actual situation.

Diana Bailey (DB): To achieve that last goal, I think it might help if we could define some sort of conceptual framework that therapists could consider when faced with dilemmas like these.

Case 1: Triage in an Elder Care Facility

DB: We thought the first case we'd talk about is the one called Triage in an Elder Care Facility. Norm, we thought that you may see some similarities between the proposed Oregon medical plan and the notion presented in this case of prioritizing clients to be treated.

Norman Daniels (ND): If you're trying to figure out how to think about this case, how much you have improved the functioning of these people, it seems to come down to this: Is going home evidence that these people are functioning on a much higher level than those who have to stay? That doesn't necessarily follow. It could be that going home simply means that these persons have more personal resources to draw on at home. In that case, the issue of "in-house" versus "out-of-house" is less informative to us. It doesn't help with the moral dimension. If we do know of a difference in functioning, it might or might not push us one way or another. But if we don't know, we have much less information on which to base the decision about triage.

Ezekiel Emanuel (EE): I have a few random thoughts on this case. The first one is that having interested relatives who are anxious to take their family members home doesn't seem to be a relevant criterion here, in part because some elderly people may not have interested family members. Or, their interested family members may not be in the same state, town, or city, and the client shouldn't be penalized because of this.

I know that in normal practice, having a relative who can either harass the therapist in the negative sense, or who in the positive sense is willing to carry on some of the work of therapy, can be an important and persuasive issue. But I think from the perspective of justice, it's not relevant.

Regarding the "persuasive physicians" in this case, I would say that the appropriateness of their taking such a role depends on why they're being persuasive. If they're persuasive because it's my client and I want you to work with my client, that is an arbitrary standpoint and you should not be swayed by it. If they're persuasive because they're making an argument to you about the client's functional capacity and potential for improvement, this may well be a relevant criterion.

But the criteria here should depend on improvement in functional capacity. In-house/out-of-house, family/no family, physician advocate/no physician advocate all are things that probably should be set aside. The main objective here is to maximally improve the function of clients.

ND: Let me ask something. Do some of these clients start out worse off than others? Is there a range of disability among these clients to begin with?

DB: Yes, there is.

Relative Benefits

ND: Then, I suggest that one qualification to what Zeke [EE] just said about the crucial considerations is this: For whom can you produce the most benefit? I'd want a more finely graded way of dividing cases. You might be willing to forego some greater benefit for some clients who start out much better off to produce a lesser benefit for clients who start out worse off. For the latter group, the improvement might make a major difference in their degree of independence because of self-esteem and other factors that play a role in function. It could be that getting somebody who starts off very badly to the point where they can do self-care activities may be an absolutely fundamental contribution, more so even than producing some higher level of functioning for someone who isn't as bad off to begin with.

It's not simply how much benefit you produce, but what the benefit does for the person who is being treated, as well as where they start and where they end up compared with the others. These are all relative considerations (Box 9-2).

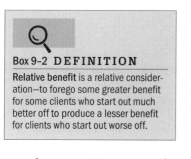

Box 9-2 DEFINITION

Relative benefit is a relative consideration—to forego some greater benefit for some clients who start out much better off to produce a lesser benefit for clients who start out worse off.

EE: Yes, there may be a threshold effect. If you start out very low, you might get over some threshold, and it may be a very important threshold. Whereas, for other people, there may be a huge increase but no major threshold that they are getting over.

Prioritizing Services

SS: Here are two questions that we've struggled with. How to prioritize improvements? For instance: Is mobility more important than cognitive capacity? How does a therapist make a judgment about that? Then, the other question has to do with "the greater good." Therapists' time is limited. So, should they spend more time with one client helping that person improve function, or do they give a little bit of time to everybody?

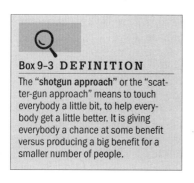

Box 9-3 DEFINITION

The "shotgun approach" or the "scatter-gun approach" means to touch everybody a little bit, to help everybody get a little better. It is giving everybody a chance at some benefit versus producing a big benefit for a smaller number of people.

DB: Yes, the "shotgun approach"— touch everybody a little bit, help everybody get a little better (Box 9-3). Or concentrate on one or two people getting a lot better. This really is the essence of rationing, isn't it?

ND: I think there's no clear answer to the question about the shotgun versus the concentration approach. Suppose all of these clients have some significant deficit in function. Then, it seems they all have a reasonable claim on the system to respond to their needs. If there are constraints here, some of the difficulty being created for occupational therapy practitioners comes from the fact that there's an inadequate supply of them.

I think it's worth acknowledging that some of the choices that have to be made in these situations shouldn't have to be made. That is, all these needs are significant; they ought to be met. Probably a lot of things we do in the healthcare system are less important than what we are talking about here. The restoration of functioning that will go on here is probably of more significant benefit for a certain number of dollars than we actually accomplish elsewhere in the healthcare system for similar money. Hard choices are being forced here because some other bad resource decisions—even unfair ones—were made elsewhere in the system.

Back to your question about whether to "give everybody a little bit" seems to respond to the idea that each person has some claim on resources. But if this means you're not accomplishing much by it, then it's not terribly valuable.

SS: That leads to my second question. How do we prioritize potential outcomes?

ND: Well, to rephrase the question: How do we rank restoration of function in different dimensions? This is probably one of the hardest questions you could ask in ethical theory. It really goes to the heart of many, many issues. And I don't think there is any brief or fully satisfactory answer.

Some methodologies purport to address this question, such as "quality of well-being" scales, or other scales that try to give an account of people's judgments about their own well-being. With these measures, we try to create a uniform scale that cuts across people's different judgments and traditions. These are riddled with all kinds of conceptual measurement problems.

For example, in Oregon, the Quality of Well-Being Scale was validated by telephoning thousands of Oregonians and asking them their feelings about having this or that health outcome (Box 9-4). The numbers that people selected didn't make any sense at all. For example, on a scale of 1 to 100 wearing eyeglasses knocks you down 5. Some people also had you lose 5 because disabilities prevented the use of public transportation.

Box 9-4 *Summary*

In Oregon, the "Quality of Well Being Scale" was validated by telephoning thousands of Oregonians and asking them their feelings about having this or that health outcome.

Does that make any sense? Perhaps this is a bad use of methodology, but my guess is that you would have to use a methodology like this several times over to get people to see the inconsistencies and to allow them to make closer decisions. Maybe then there would be some convergence in people's views about which kinds of conditions or losses of function are worse than which others. My guess is that we don't have the methodologies for doing that. Nor do we have a set of principles that you can appeal to that would let you say so much loss of mobility is always worse than so much loss of some other function.

DB: Don't you think that would vary from person to person, so it wouldn't make sense to try to standardize it in that way?

ND: It might make sense to have some standard measurements because you might need such a list for certain kinds of resource allocation questions. But in terms of what it's worth for a particular client or what a particular client wants done, it would be the client's own assessment of the relative importance of these goals.

Suppose you pose the question from within the perspective of one person. You can get a clearer answer. The person can say, "I have a choice. I can work on being able to feed myself, or I can work on being able to dress myself." The therapist would say, "Which would be more important for you to try to do first?" And the person might answer, "The most important to me is that I don't want anybody to have to help me in the bathroom. That's the most important thing. Other things, I'll work on later." Then you're getting a clear answer.

Some people may have different judgments around these issues. So, if what therapists have to allocate is time, then they can get a more finely graded answer about what to do with their time in consultation with the client. What they want to do reflects what the client wants— what is most important to the client in that situation. This is a way for the client to convert the therapist's time into an outcome for that client.

EE: The problem of the case that we are presented with here, however, is a little different. The problem is the interpersonal comparison between the treatment one person gets versus what another person gets. That's much more difficult and, as I think Norm correctly points out, we don't have a standard that we agree works well.

SS: Let's say the therapist has a client who was a professor, who has cognitive problems and wants to work on memory skills. Another person may have been a construction worker and may prefer to be more independent in mobility. What do therapists do when they have time to treat only one of them? If both clients have equal potential to achieve?

EE: I think one of the questions you want to ask in these kinds of comparisons is: What kind of change are you going to produce for these people? Is it possible in either situation to create a major move in independence in that particular sphere? Also, how debilitating is their condition for these people? These judgments are crude and somewhat intuitive, but they do have appeal to some ethical standards that we understand.

Again, I think the problem of the shotgun approach is that it's not going to give anyone sufficient attention to really make a major difference, and you don't want to dissipate your energy. You want to have people improve in a significant way, so being more focused does have its appeal.

I think it's important for therapists to recognize that these are ethical choices within a larger system, where the larger system itself has systemic injustices. Occupational therapy practitioners alone can't be responsible for these injustices.

ND: I do think, though, that you're not going to be able to come up with an ordering or priority for improving cognitive function versus improving mobility versus something else. A more reasonable approach for the therapist would be to say, "Well, how much time do I have? If I take so many units of my time and use them on this client versus that client, what could the different outcomes be for those clients? I must also have some input from those clients about what's more important to them. This is a multifactored judgment about how to allocate my time. I should try to capture several dimensions of thinking and be responsive to what's most important from the client's point of view, and to produce enough benefit to make a real change."

Family Needs

SS: We often have families who get involved in their family member's treatment, of course, and the client's level of independence affects the family—making the client less dependent on the family. Is that something you judge important?

EE: Yes, indeed. People don't want to be dependent. For example, having to have your daughter take you to the bathroom may be very demeaning, more demeaning even than having an attendant or someone outside the family do it. So that may be a relevant criterion. Not because the family wants the clients not to be dependent, but because the client him- or herself views this independence as an important outcome.

DB: Another situation is when the family says, "If my family member cannot be independent in toileting, I cannot care for him in my home." So in this case, the decision might revolve around the family's needs rather than the client's.

ND: Not necessarily. The family says, "Look, we're happy to take this person home, but we can't deal with toileting. So, if you've got to make a choice about which task to concentrate on, then concentrate on toileting and we'll help the client deal with other things." So, what's the loss to the client if that choice, in effect, gets forced on the client by the family? Is there something else the client would have preferred working on? There may or may not be. The client might say, "Ideally I would rather have worked on mobility, but I don't want to be in this facility. I want to be with my family, and if that's what it takes, then that's what it takes." So what's the loss?

Prioritizing Care and Third-Party Payors

EE: In another portion of the case, we are asked who should be prioritized—those likely to return home soonest or those who could increase their independence quickly while remaining in the facility?

ND: That's a good question. I'm not sure I know enough to be able to give a clear answer. Suppose it's a priority of certain third-party payors to get people out of facilities as quickly as possible, which is likely the case in a managed care facility (Box 9-5). Then, somebody else is setting the priority. Now the issue for the therapist is: "How do I abide by these priorities when I think they might be harming the interests of certain other clients?"

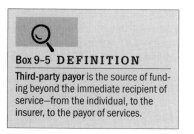

Box 9-5 DEFINITION

Third-party payor is the source of funding beyond the immediate recipient of service—from the individual, to the insurer, to the payor of services.

That's more likely the form the question really takes for the therapist than the way you put it here [in the case]. The question is: What is being lost for certain clients if the priority must be getting people out quickly, so as to keep costs down?

SS: Then the priority would go to the healthiest, the people who have the best outcome according to someone else's criteria?

EE: I think this goes back to the issue of merely going home, which is not in itself an independence marker that should be valued by the therapist. Just the fact that a client can go home—and that's of interest to the administration for financial reasons—does not constitute the driving force that should govern the therapist.

SS: How do we know what the therapist should be thinking about? Where does that judgment come from?

EE: I think that the therapist's primary obligation is to his or her clients and to help them gain functional improvement.

DB: Not to the government, to third-party payors, or to the institution?

EE: Not to the third-party payors. What they view as most important is what's going to generate the most profit for them. I just don't think that's the therapist's motive. Occasionally, motives will be in conflict, and I think that therapists have to be aware of this possibility. There are other more subtle cases in which there may be similar problems for them. For example, facilities are frequently full, and getting new clients who can benefit from treatment is a problem. This can happen only when you discharge clients by getting them to suitably independent function.

Obligation to Potential Clients

ND: Now here's an interesting problem because Linda [in the case] actually has clients now, and the question is, what is her obligation to potential clients? They're not her clients yet.

DB: Does she have an obligation to those potential clients?

EE: I think she has an obligation, but it's not as strong as her obligation to her actual clients. This issue revolves around systemic problems, in terms of production of suitable numbers of occupational and physical therapists. Linda can't be solely responsible for the existence of a suitable number of beds in rehabilitation facilities, and so on. But that isn't to say that she has zero obligation to think about the future stream of clients into her facility. I think she does have some obligation. For her to focus her energies on people who aren't going to make a significant improvement, to break a threshold might not be a good judgment. Again, I think that obligation is not strong, not powerful, especially if she is incurring a lot of benefit for current clients. But I don't think it's nonexistent.

ND: I think there's another background consideration in connection with third-party payors wanting to lower costs. This has a lot to do with background beliefs about the overall fairness of the system. If you think a decision to lower costs is a way to most effectively use resources in various parts of the system, then you may want to respect it more. But if you think the motivation is to improve the bottom line of this company and nobody is considering where to steer the resources saved, you may not want to consider it very carefully.

Helping Therapists Make Choices

SS: How does this therapist make these decisions? Does she do it alone or does she try to involve the administration? Does she do it regardless of what her supervisor says if she believes she's made the right decision?

EE: I think these are two different questions. One is what you would try to do within the system to shift the system at your facility in a certain direction. For example, perhaps they could hire more therapists, possibly part-time, and you could be involved in petitioning the administration or your supervisor to consider this solution.

The second question is how do you choose your particular clients if you can't satisfy all of them? This question goes back to the comments we were making at the start. I think a blanket view—I'm going to help only the healthiest who can get out or I'm going to help only those who are the worst off here and have multiple problems—is probably not the best view to take. But it may be that for those worst-off clients, you might be able to make some significant changes, even if they're not going to be independent; then that is suitable and justifiable.

DB: Significant. The therapist has to be able to decide what is a significant change?

EE: Yes, but at this stage of the game we don't have a criterion on which we can uniformly rely and find justifiable, either as a society or philosophically. Therefore, to try to hold off these decisions until we get that kind of ranking is not practical. Therapists are going to be involved in these types of decisions now.

Prioritizing Sick/Sicker Clients for Treatment

ND: I think you have to temper the decision about worse-off clients versus healthier clients by some judgment about what degree of benefit you can produce within each category. In some ways I agree with the concern about helping the worst off and giving them some priority or claim to services, but not if you can produce only minuscule benefits for them while others are foregoing very significant benefits. So you have to factor into your judgment about best-off/worst-off clients some assessment of likely outcome for each category. We don't have refined rules that tell you how to make those judgments.

EE: This isn't unique to occupational therapy.

ND: I think it is one of the unsolved moral problems in the rationing of health care. It is the issue of how much priority you give the sickest people and how much benefit for others you would be willing to sacrifice to produce benefits for the worst-off groups. We don't have a principled way of answering this question.

Another question that we don't have a principled way of answering is embedded in the "scatter-gun approach"—giving everybody a chance at some benefit versus producing the biggest benefit for a smaller number of people. This is a case of giving a fair chance of some improvement to all versus favoring the best outcomes when allocating resources. It's a problem we don't know how to answer. It's not just in health care; these problems show up in other places in life, too. So the issues you're touching on here have the structure of classic problems, but the bad news is that they're unsolved.

SS: But we have to make practical decisions.

ND: Yes, you have to make practical decisions. My inclination—to go to the issue of process—is to try to involve more people and develop a clear statement for the reasons you're making your choices. Get some input from others working in the institution about why you're inclined to do it one way over another. They may have good suggestions about why it's bad, or you may bring out the bad suggestions—say, for purely financial reasons—and so on. That's the downside of opening the process up and making it less professional. My sense is that you might be able to reduce tension and the burden on the individual decision maker if you can create a climate in which people see these as difficult decisions that don't have a good clean, clear answer. Then, maybe they will tolerate some range of approaches.

Case 2: Too Many Cases to Handle

DB: Can we move to another case that brings in what Norm was just saying about trying to involve as many people as possible in the decision. In "Too Many Cases to Handle," where Julio is going out into the community to work with a person whose reputation is as a drug dealer, should Julio be making that decision? Should he be deciding whether to continue treatment, or should his supervisor be making the decision, or should it be an even higher management decision?

EE: I was a little frustrated by this case because there are a lot of choices to be made and the context isn't completely clear. For example, it says, "If he documents some minor improvements." Well, are there minor improvements or not? Or even major improvements? It appears that we aren't at the stage where those are likely; the time frame for evaluation has been too short.

Let's assume the best-case scenario: that there are some changes and there is the anticipation of some more significant changes, not just in the narrow focus, but also potentially in the larger focus of this guy getting drug rehabilitation services. There is clearly also the systemic pressure of the facility threatening to cut off funds. This does seem to be a case in which enlisting other people who are involved in the case (although not directly)—your supervisor, any social work advocates who might be available—does seem to be a useful approach.

If we're talking about straightforward lying, where there's no improvement . . .

DB: I think that's the implication.

EE: Yes, the case does suggest to me that there's no improvement, and the hope for improvement is probably minimal. The reason for involvement here is that the therapist has a good rapport with the client and he might get him into drug rehabilitation. The therapist is going to lie for that? Uh, uh. I find that not really justifiable. Julio is an occupational therapist. Whereas his concern is with the client in a large sense, he's not the custodian or guardian for this person.

"Gaming" the System

ND: So your point is that it's not really the therapist's role? Whereas you might tolerate "gaming" the system for some benefit that is within Julio's professional capacity and where he could see a reasonable prospect of some good happening? The problem here is getting the client into drug rehab.

EE: No one denies that drug counseling might be good for this person. To achieve that, it might be more legitimate to "game" the system.

ND: So yours was not a hard-and-fast rule against "gaming" a third-party payor [laughter], but you wanted it to be done within some reasonable constraint regarding the professional roles of this person?

EE: That's one constraint. I think another constraint is what you actually have to do to "game" the system—to outright lie. If this is a case where there is no improvement and you have to say there is improvement to continue and your hope of improvement is small, then you're really going out on a limb.

ND: But that's only to say there's less justification for lying.

EE: Also, the lie is bigger. [Laughter]

ND: The point is that if there are small changes, then you're not lying. The only case in which there is a choice here is if there aren't any documented changes, but you think there are likely to be some.

Then you stall them by lying to get the benefit for the client. This seems to be okay. What you're saying is you can't lie if the benefit is not an occupational therapy benefit, but it's getting the client into drug rehab. Then it's drug therapy, not occupational therapy.

DB: This is not an uncommon problem, this issue of there being a hiatus with no improvement, but we can clearly expect that there will be some improvement in a week or two, and therapists constantly make this judgment. Do I lie and document some sort of minor improvement in the anticipation that, with legitimate treatment techniques, there will be a great deal of improvement down the line? So maybe we could talk about it from that perspective.

ND: The point is that insurers have this rule, that if there's no change then this is just custodial care and therefore everything else is out. This is a very bureaucratic rule to start with. It doesn't allow for fine judgments, where benefit will be just around the corner. In the spirit of saying that the rule is really just too crude to deal with delivering appropriate benefits, you might have some justification for saying, "Well, you know, the rule is only an approximation, and I'm going to approximate in a different way." And that's not exactly . . . I wouldn't consider that . . . cheating.

DB: Then it's not a lie. [Laughter]

EE: I think there are cases where you'd provide therapy for a certain amount of time and you could say 20 percent of people will respond. You provide it for longer, 50 percent; you provide it for even longer, 70 percent. Where you draw that cutoff can be extremely arbitrary and bureaucratic. And this may be such a case, "We'll give you 4 weeks, no improvement, end it." Whereas you might expect only 50 percent of people to respond in the 4 weeks and a good portion to respond shortly thereafter.

These are the kinds of cases where, call it lying, call it "gaming" the system, call it trying to get the best for the client, but arguing with the payor that this is a case where you have reasons to expect improvement is a good idea. These are the cases where you want to be more forceful about it.

In my experience in oncology and talking to drug companies (it may be slightly different talking to insurance companies for you), when you do activate the system, it doesn't tend to be a lie. You're not saying, "Yes, there was a dramatic change," or even "there was a change," but rather, "I want to try for X amount longer, and here are the reasons."

Is This a Dilemma?

SS: Would you go so far as to say that there is no dilemma here? Because one of the things that Diana and I have talked about is when it is that something really becomes a dilemma.

EE: My problem with this case is that there is insufficient background material for me to know. But I think you can construct a situation in which, what appears initially to be an ethical problem soon evaporates. If there are minor changes, you can push the insurance company around a little bit. But if you have to outright lie when there's been no improvement and the anticipation of improvement is not very high, I do think that's wrong. I don't think there's justification.

My experience with insurers is that they tend to be less "hard and fast" than this. There are rules about the number of weeks the therapy can go on, but those rules are loose, and pushing them for good reason may work. Again, I'm hesitant to say that in this case there is good reason.

Case 1: Triage in an Elder Care Facility

SS: Now, could you clarify what would make the other case more of a dilemma? The triage situation in the elder care facility: in what sense is that clearly an ethical dilemma?

EE: There, you actually have groups of clients, all of whom are going to receive benefit—benefit that you can directly bring them—and you may be forced because of the allocation of your time to choose between them. This seems to me to be a very clear dilemma.

Actually there are two dilemmas. First, you're forced to choose between particular clients, both of whom can benefit. Second, you may be forced to compare benefits that seem incommensurate to you, at least at first glance. Mobility versus dressing improvements, for instance, where you're not sure how to weigh them. We're pretty sure we don't know how to weigh them, at least at this point in our philosophical progress.

Unsafe Work Environments

DB: What are the issues that should be considered when a healthcare worker is expected to visit a client's home that may be unsafe, or one that is in an unsafe area? Is there an ethical dilemma there?

EE: Certainly one of prudence.

ND: Well, no, there's more. I mean, it's like the analogue, I suppose, for the AIDS situation. How much risk is part of your job? What is the standard? There's probably not a very clear answer to that situation. Somebody who accepted the role of therapist in an area where it was common to have to go to inner-city areas or to work with people in housing projects presumably had a certain amount of choice. If this is the job and this is the clientele for people who have this job, my view is your consent to accepting those risks would be your agreement to be in this job. If you say, "I won't go to these places," then it would seem to me that the person running this clinic could say, "Well, I guess you won't be able to work for us. You go find another job where you will feel comfortable."

This is a situation in which a person is making a choice: "Do I want to take these risks or don't I?" But suppose somebody says, "I'm willing to accept the general location, but certain places are especially dangerous, and I don't want to go to those." Then I think it's unfair to ask a therapist to go to those places without someone going with them or without some special protections.

Case 3: The Seven-Day Work Week

SS: I wonder if we could look at the case of the nursing staff being asked to do activities in the occupational therapy room in the evenings? In some settings, because there is not enough money to pay an occupational therapist, administrators will say, "We have nursing staff here in the evening, let them do occupational therapy." But, of course, they're not occupational therapists, and it leaves therapists in a quandary about refusing to give the nurses therapy supplies, because they're seen as withholding. But the nurses are not trained to be selective about which activities are appropriate for the clients.

This issue is tied in with the therapists' not being in the facility in the evening. Therapists used to provide care 9 A.M. to 5 P.M., 5 days a week. Now they're being asked to provide services weekends and evenings. Because there is insufficient staff, therapists are being stretched. There is insufficient money to hire additional staff; otherwise, if they had somebody to work evenings and weekends, the therapist, in Aruzhana's case, wouldn't have a problem.

Is This Occupational Therapy?

ND: So the facility wants to give the nurses the materials and have the nurses play with the clients because they don't really know how to treat them with activities. What will the facility do? Charge for occupational therapy, even though it's not occupational therapy? What is their interest in claiming that this is occupational therapy?

SS: Because then they fulfill their contracts with the insurers.

What Should Aruzhana Do?

ND: I think Aruzhana should refuse. I think this is a real case of lowering professional standards to meet the financial requirements. What is being done here should not count in your financial contract, or in any other way, as occupational therapy. The administration is trying to cheat. They'll just have to hire some other therapists. You can't have it both ways.

SS: So this is not really an ethical dilemma?

EE: No, it isn't. There's an answer!

ND: That's how I see it, too. I would see this as a danger in some managed care practices. They say, "Well, the benefit package will include occupational therapy." What does that mean when it comes to the managed care arrangement—is this client going to get treated by occupational therapists? Not if this managed care facility has anything to do with it; they'll get the materials handed out by a nurse! That's not occupational therapy, so let's call it what it is and say, "This is the wrong thing to do. This is an unreasonable compromise. It would be unprofessional for me to permit something to be called treatment, when it really isn't treatment."

EE: I think Aruzhana has the advantage in this case. On the one hand, she says that there are certain tools of the trade—like a surgeon giving the scalpel to a nurse—that's not the activity. On the other hand, she's saying that certain activities can act as bridges, which aren't specifically occupational therapy. Like the recreational program, which is not an occupational therapy program, but is for the clients' benefit. So I see it as a bridge.

I think the idea of making Aruzhana work new extended hours is a contract negotiation issue, because the duties of her job are being redefined.

Going back to the first issue, I presume an evaluation would go along with the activity's use, if an occupational therapist were using it. So there is an issue here of individual versus group treatment. If these clients can realize benefit in a group setting and that benefit is important, it may be fine. But if the only way they can gain measurable improvement is through individual therapy—and the group setting is really more for the administration than therapy for the clients—then it's wrong.

I think the objective has to be the client. There could be a conflict in which a person could get a lot of benefit in a group setting, but could also get benefit in an individual setting and time doesn't permit you to have both. This may be a dilemma that isn't easily resolved.

SS: The situation of treating the client who has senile dementia, for example, and who wanders, and may need one-to-one attention from the therapist. The therapist has to make a decision. Does she see eight people in a group because the reimbursement will be greater, or does she spend time with this one individual who may have a better outcome as an individual? How do you compare the outcome for an individual with the outcome for a group?

EE: We don't have a general answer to that question. I think Norm is right. On the other hand, if this could be a significant benefit for the individual and the group of eight is just an enrichment program, in which we're not expecting any major improvements, we may easily justify care for that one person.

DB: I see we have run out of time. Sharan and I want to thank you for taking an hour from your busy schedules for this project. This discussion has really increased our understanding of the issues involved in rationing treatment and helped us formulate several ways to examine these issues. Concepts such as relative benefits, prioritizing services, concerns with third-party reimbursers, family versus client desires, and group versus individual treatment should be considered in discussing dilemmas to decide on a plan of action.

Study Questions

1. Identify three criteria for determining which clients "deserve" priority for occupational therapy services.

2. Under what circumstances should occupational therapists deny services to clients?

3. When does rationing of occupational therapy services move from unethical to illegal?

4. How or by what standards can occupational therapists determine fees in relation to caseload and reimbursement practices?

5. Can quality of life be measured objectively? By what means and for what purposes? What are the hazards of solely using objective measures for functional outcomes?

6. Read the following case and apply Hansen and Kyler-Hutchinson's (1992) questions to resolution of the dilemma:

   a. Who are the players?
   b. What other facts or information are needed?
   c. What are the possible actions that could be taken?
   d. What are the likely consequences of each action?
   e. Choose an action you can defend.

Insurance Dictating Treatment

Gary Bernstein, OTR, has been treating Mrs. Jaycynski for 8 weeks in the rehabilitation department of a large rehabilitation facility. Mrs. Jaycynski has made remarkable progress since her cerebrovascular accident but appears to have reached a plateau for the moment. Mr. Bernstein has 9 years of experience working with clients with conditions such as Mrs. Jaycynski's, and he is sure that she will make more progress in therapy in another week or so.

Mrs. Jaycynski's insurance company states that if no progress can be shown at the end of each week, therapy will no longer be paid for and should cease. Mr. Bernstein is tempted to document continued progress for this week even though this is not strictly true, so that reimbursement can continue. Once reimbursement has terminated for a condition/illness, it cannot be restarted. Mr. Bernstein would like Mrs. Jaycynski to have the opportunity to receive occupational therapy for the next 2 to 3 weeks because he is sure she will improve more. Is Mr. Bernstein justified is falsifying this week's progress note in the client's chart?

Patient Rights: Informed Consent, Competence, and the Right to Refuse Treatment

CASE 1: Bipolar Disorder and ARC

CASE 2: Family Imposes Treatment on Relative

with commentaries by **Thomas G. Gutheil, MD,** *and* **Penny Kyler, MA, OTR, FAOTA**

Key Terms

Competence
Guardian
Informed consent

Informed consent emergencies
Specific competence

CASE 1: Bipolar Disorder and ARC

You are currently working in a state psychiatric hospital, and one patient on your unit is diagnosed with bipolar disorder and acquired immunodeficiency syndrome (AIDS)-related complex (ARC). The patient has a long history of bipolar disorder and is a frequent visitor to the state hospital.

During previous manic episodes, the patient has shown aggression toward other patients and staff. Currently, she has escalated into a hypermanic phase that is associated with hypersexism, poor insight, and loss of control. She has been smearing blood and other body fluids on the walls of her room and is threatening patients and staff with the same.

The staff has a long list of questions and concerns. The following are two important questions: (1) What are this patient's rights, especially related to confidentiality, seclusion, and the use of restraints? and (2) What are the rights of the other patients, staff, and visitors?

CASE 2: Family Imposes Treatment on Relative

Mrs. Ciarrelli has early-stage Alzheimer's disease, and her son and daughter-in-law and their children live with her in her home. Her son and daughter-in-law both work, and the children are at school, which leaves Mrs. Ciarrelli at home alone all day Monday through Friday. Mrs. Ciarrelli sometimes becomes confused, forgets to eat, and starts activities and leaves them unfinished because she forgets what she is doing. She has occasionally engaged in unsafe behavior such as putting on the kettle and forgetting it, and walking downstairs with her bathrobe belt undone and dangling around her legs.

Although she is basically safe at the moment, the Ciarrellis feel certain that Mrs. Ciarrelli could benefit from occupational therapy under home health services (her insurance would pay for such a service). An occupational therapist could ensure that she prepares herself a nutritious lunch and uses her time productively and safely. Mrs. Ciarrelli, however, wants no part of occupational therapy. She does not want a stranger coming into her home "telling her what to do."

Should she be "forced" to receive occupational therapy as a result of her family deeming her incompetent to make that decision?

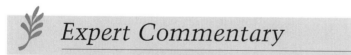

Expert Commentary

by Thomas G. Gutheil, MD

In the past, mentally ill persons, particularly those incarcerated in institutions, forfeited many of their rights. Recent decades have seen the definition and elaboration of the rights of patients in several different areas of social life. This chapter addresses some of these rights issues and the theories underlying them.

Informed Consent

A useful starting point is the central notion of **informed consent**. Until relatively recently, physicians were expected to tell patients about their

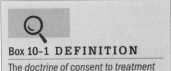

Box 10-1 DEFINITION

The *doctrine of consent to treatment* states that physicians planning a treatment regimen or surgical procedure must obtain a patient's consent to do so; otherwise, the doctor is committing a battery, an unconsented touching.

Box 10-2 *Summary*

To be meaningful, a patient's consent must be informed so that decisions can be made in a reasoned manner.

illnesses only what the physician deemed fit. This medical paternalism was fairly standard. Earlier in the twentieth century, the doctrine of consent to treatment was articulated. Physicians planning a treatment regimen or surgical procedure had to obtain the patient's consent to do so; otherwise, the doctor was committing a battery, an unconsented touching (Box 10-1).

Recent developments articulated the principle that simple consent or "yeasaying" was insufficient to respect the patient's right to autonomy over what would happen to the patient's body. To be meaningful, the patient's consent had to be informed, so that the decision could be made in a reasoned manner (Box 10-2).

Competence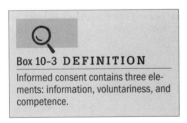

Note that the theoretical model—a well-informed patient thoughtfully and rationally making a decision by carefully weighing the issues—does not apply in many cases. Like most other decisions in human affairs, treatment decisions are actually made by a combination of intuition, visceral instincts, and trust within the relationship with the caretaker. These issues become even more convoluted when the patient is acutely ill or when the patient's decision-making capability is impaired because of the underlying illness at which the treatment in question is aimed.

Nevertheless, the formal doctrine of informed consent assumes rational decision making by a knowledgeable decision maker. Informed consent now contains three elements: information, voluntariness, and competence (Box 10-3).

Under the rubric of *information,* an established universe of data is expected to be conveyed by the doctor to the patient for purposes of the patient's decision making. This information includes the risks and benefits of the proposed treatment; the risks and benefits of alternative treatments that might also be appropriate to treat the problem in question; and the risks and benefits (or consequences) of leaving the illness untreated, that is, the results of no treatment.

Box 10-3 DEFINITION

Informed consent contains three elements: information, voluntariness, and competence.

Voluntariness is the "consent" in informed consent. Coercion to treatment or threats if the plan is not followed are obvious examples of infringement of the voluntariness of the decision. The alternative face of voluntary acceptance of treatment is the refusal of treatment (see description on the right to refuse treatment).

Competence refers to the individual's capacity to weigh the information in processing the decision. If this capacity is present, a competent patient may (1) reject even life-saving treatment, (2) embark on even a very risky research treatment protocol with an experimental drug, (3) accept a treatment plan with a very poor likelihood of success, and (4) agree to take a medication, for instance, for a purpose different from that for which the medication was originally used. To illustrate the last point, carbamazepine is an anticonvulsant that has proven to be exceptionally useful in manic-depressive illness and that has been extensively researched and described in the clinical literature; however, it is still described in drug companies' package inserts and in the *Physicians' Desk Reference* only as an anticonvulsant. A competent patient may give informed consent to such use.

It may not be immediately obvious, but the capacity to weigh the risks and benefits of a treatment to consent to it is identical with the capacity to do the same and to decide to refuse it. The "yes" and "no" in this decision are two sides of the same coin.

The Emergency Exception

An emergency situation represents an exception to the rule that informed consent must be obtained for treatment interventions. Emergencies are recognized as special circumstances in which certain rules must be suspended to save life or prevent acute injury, deterioration, or similar harm (Box 10-4). Some typical interventions permitted only under emergency conditions are breach of confidentiality, involuntary treatment, and involuntary hospitalization (commitment). The question of treatment against a patient's will in nonemergency conditions is discussed in the following section.

Box 10-4 *By the Law*

An emergency situation represents an exception to the rule that informed consent must be obtained for treatment interventions. **Informed consent emergencies** are special circumstances in which certain rules must be suspended to save a life or prevent acute injury, deterioration, or similar harm.

The *Right to Refuse Treatment*

Until the mid- to late 1970s, commitment of mentally ill patients was presumed to permit treatment of the patient even against his or her will. This was done because confinement without treatment would simply be considered impermissible incarceration. Of concern to health practitioners would be the type of commitment that provided no pathway for eventual release through treatment of the underlying illness that had occasioned the confinement. The patient's refusal of treatment, if any, was not honored because it was presumed to flow from the same impaired decision making that prompted refusal of hospitalization, which in turn had necessitated the commitment. In addition, the presumed dangerousness of the patient—an essential justification for the confinement—also played some conceptual role in justifying the treatment of a patient against his or her will.

In the subsequent turbulent decade, many social movements addressed the rights of oppressed, disenfranchised, or powerless populations such as minorities, prisoners, and, comparably, the mentally ill. One of the byproducts of these movements in the legal context surrounding the mentally ill was the separation of treatment from commitment as if it were a separate issue: the so-called commitment/treatment schism.

As mental health case law evolved, commitment of patients began to be justifiable only by dangerousness and not, as before, by the need for treatment; commitment and treatment could be thus theoretically separated: commitment was for the protection of society, whereas treatment was a separate issue, rendered less urgent anyway because the patient was "behind bars." Clinicians were puzzled because they understood clearly how the patient's rejection of hospitalization as treatment usually sprang from the *same* psychological wellspring as refusal of other treatments. Hence, this separation between the two issues appeared artificial and clinically unrealistic.

For precision, note that the particular treatment representing the major focus of the extensive literature, case law, legislation, and debate was the treatment of psychosis with antipsychotic medication. Although in theory all treatments are presumed to fall under the conceptual heading of "the right to refuse," the treatments whose refusal is under discussion usually consist of these useful, effective, although uncomfortable drugs. The complexity of these issues cannot be more extensively addressed here; the reader is referred to other sources (see Additional Reading).

Under the reasoning of the commitment/treatment schism, the dangerousness of the patient was replaced as a critical factor by the question of the patient's competence to consent to (or refuse) treatment. There is an undeniable logic to this rationale: Only those inpatients capable of giving informed consent would receive treatment. But there, it rapidly emerged, was the rub: What if the patient was, indeed, not competent to consent?

The usual response to incompetence in a given individual was guardianship, a tradition extensively rooted in English and subsequent American law (Box 10-5). The guardian—in former times appointed by the king, but more recently by a judge—would act as vicarious decision maker on behalf of the incompetent person, called the ward. For the indigent state hospital population, however, often allied with absent,

Box 10-5 *Summary*

One response to incompetence in a given individual is to assign a **guardian** who acts as a vicarious decision maker on behalf of the incompetent person.

avoidant, or dysfunctional families, the supply of potential guardians was nearly nonexistent.

In a variation on this theme, some jurisdictions required a judicial hearing, with full legal panoply, to decide whether a refusing patient could be made to accept medications. Empirical evidence reveals that this mechanism is not only the most expensive, cumbersome, and time consuming, but also the least effective at honoring patients' refusals! It remains to be seen what other developments will occur in this area.

In the present era, this once hotly debated issue has decayed into procedure. Most jurisdictions that have experienced (or are fearing to experience) a lawsuit on this issue have developed standardized rules and protocols for responding to a patient's questionably competent refusal of treatment.

Other Rights of Patients

For completeness, note that other rights commonly seen on lists of this topic (e.g., on "bills of rights" established by healthcare organizations and facilities) are rights to privacy, to correspondence and communication by phone or mail, to a safe environment and certain standards of facility and staffing, to visitation, to confidentiality, to legal consultation, and to dignity (Box 10-6). This list may vary regionally, but the items noted are common and widely used in defining the rights that patients, although hospitalized, retain.

> **Box 10-6 *Summary***
>
> Rights for patients who are hospitalized are usually thought to include the right to accept or reject treatment based on sufficient information, rights to privacy, to correspondence and communication by phone or mail, to a safe environment and certain standards of facility and staffing, to visitation, to confidentiality, to legal consultation, and to dignity.

Case Scenarios

With the preceding background to orient us, let us consider the case examples. The case example "Bipolar Disorder and ARC" captures the complexity of professionals' often-competing legal and ethical duties to individual inpatients in tension with duties to other patients and to the milieu as a whole (Box 10-7). The patient is described as escalating to being out of control and smearing body fluids (now rendered dangerous instead of merely messy by the diagnosis of ARC). The situation clearly justifies labeling as an emergency in both a literal and an affective sense, as well as a danger for predictable further escalation if mania is not controlled. The patient should be secluded or restrained by as many staff members as are needed for safety and treatment, involun-

> **Box 10-7 *Ethical Dilemma***
>
> The first scenario captures the complexity of a professional's often-competing legal and ethical duties to individual inpatients in tension with duties to other patients and to the milieu as a whole.

tarily. When more controlled and stable, the patient should be encouraged to explore her behavior and its possible consequences.

The question becomes more complex in relation to the rights of other patients, staff, and visitors. First, the use of Universal Precautions, a nondiscriminatory approach based on an assumption that everyone may have the human immunodeficiency virus (HIV) and using protections accordingly, honors rights of privacy by not discriminating against, and thus identifying, patients with this disease in some form. Most jurisdictions give first consideration to the right of confidentiality about AIDS and its accompaniments.

Staff members need to perform a dangerousness assessment of this patient just as if the threats were of violence rather than infection; the response to the patient would then be dictated by the patient's condition, as always. A conservative response—not letting the lack of control escalate very far before intervening—is recommended. Keep in mind that other patients on the ward are a captive audience and deserve protection as well. Although not all accidents or encounters are foreseeable or preventable, efforts in this direction should be made.

The patient's right to receive visitors has a discretionary aspect; that is, it may be suspended for good cause (which should be explicitly documented). In this case, visitors would be restricted and turned away. Visitors have the right to some protection, and a patient's clinical ability to tolerate visitation should be determined by staff and a decision made about visiting. Some visitors might be selectively restricted if they are found to escalate the patient, bring in contraband, and so forth.

Box 10-8 *Ethical Dilemma*

A useful approach to dealing with confidentiality concerning AIDS-related issues is to have the patient himself or herself pass on the information to specific others such as family, partner, or spouse.

A useful approach to dealing with confidentiality concerning AIDS-related issues is to have the patient pass on the information to specific others such as family, partner, or spouse (Box 10-8). The patient has no professional obligation to maintain confidentiality; hence, he or she may be persuaded to inform others. If the patient is willing, this approach may solve many of the problems arising from such a patient's presence on a ward.

The case of Mrs. Ciarrelli, "Family Imposes Treatment on Relative," presents a different set of concerns. Both Mrs. Ciarrelli's functional capacity and her competence have been rendered suspect because of her Alzheimer's disease. Hence, her refusal of occupational therapy may be similarly suspect.

In this case, the occupational therapist may play an extremely valuable but uncustomary role—"case finder." The family, together with physician and attorney, if possible, might bring Mrs. Ciarrelli's case before the Probate Court in her jurisdiction for an assessment of her competency to make decisions about her welfare and safety. If Mrs. Ciarrelli is found competent, efforts may be required to deal with her potential dangerousness by institutionalization in some form. If she is found incompetent, the guardian (who might be a family member or attorney or other) would be empowered to make the decision—in this case, about occupational therapy.

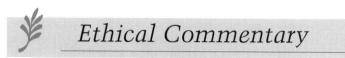

Ethical Commentary

by Penny Kyler, MA, OTR, FAOTA

Case 1: Bipolar Disorder and ARC

In this scenario, concerns in mental health practice have been presented. Although occupational therapy has its roots in mental health, the problems that practitioners face today are different from those faced by practitioners in the 1940s and 1950s. Treatment is compounded by issues concerning confidentiality, the possibility of litigation, social issues such as homelessness, and lack of work opportunities. Partly because of these concerns, occupational therapy practitioners working in either inpatient or community facilities still have an important role to play in the treatment of persons with chronic mental disorders.

Who Are the Players?

The players are the patient with bipolar disorder and ARC, her family, other patients, visitors, staff at the hospital, the patients' rights advocate, clinical departments, and the hospital ethics committee. Are there any others?

What Other Information Is Needed?

How have this patient's previous hospitalizations progressed? Has she exhibited the same behavior? Is the patient considered mentally competent? Is there a family member or friend who can successfully communicate with her? Is there a particular staff person with whom this patient has a good relationship? Is there a hospital ethics committee? What is the hospital policy on patient confidentiality? What are the policies on infection control and the use of Universal Precautions? What type of medication has been prescribed? Are there other questions?

What Actions May Be Taken and What Are the Possible Consequences?

In this case scenario, those in charge of the patient's treatment need to consider several issues. The issue of confidentiality has been thoroughly discussed by Dr. Gutheil. Another issue is that of an assessment. This patient should receive an assessment to determine possible organic impairment before the practitioner decides on a course of action. Such an assessment would provide the physician with information that would probably help shape the treatment approach. The assessment would also determine the patient's ability to understand the implications of ARC.

A patient with bipolar disease may willingly share information when the disease is controlled and may refuse to share information when in a hypermanic phase. Staff members will have to deal with this difficulty when trying to elicit the health status of this patient. There may also be the need for occupational therapy staff members to determine what goal-directed activities may be done with the patient alone or in groups and how these activities may affect the usual process of occupational therapy with other patients.

The risk of HIV infection is primarily limited to intimate contact with exchange of body fluids. Such an event is possible within the hospital, and the first consideration must be that of saving lives. Would sharing confidential information with the ward community save lives? The duty of staff members to protect other patients is paramount. Along with the usual medication and seclusion routine, an ongoing AIDS education program should be part of the patient education program at the hospital.

A patient who is in the midst of a psychotic episode cries out for the paternalistic model of health care to be used; however, we have moved away from this model of care to client-centered care. Physicians often adopt one of several models for their client-centered interactions with patients, including (1) the *informative model* that assumes a clear distinction between facts provided by the physician and the patient's values; (2) the *interpretive model* where the physician helps the patient articulate his or her values in determining the medical interventions; and (3) the *deliberative model* where the physician discusses health-related values that are affected by the patient's disease or treatment (Emanual & Emanual, 1992). The important distinction between the models is the physician's role as technical expert, teacher, guardian, or advisor and how this role affects the patient's autonomy.

An important question here is whether any of these models can be used with this hypermanic patient. Or would using a paternalistic model be preferable because it would place the patient's medical interests and the interests of others in the community in the forefront? And finally, would prescribing medication and revisiting these issues in 72 hours be a better course of action?

Case 2: Family Imposes Treatment on Relative

In some cultures, elders are venerated for their wisdom, and it is accepted that those who live beyond the sixth decade are deserving of some latitude. This latitude is often played out in the ability of individuals to have their routine daily life tasks undisturbed by the younger people involved in the elders' lives. Our culture in the United States, however, has moved to a point where we find it difficult to leave elders managing on their own, particularly when the caregivers are unsure of the elders' safety. Principle 1.A of the occupational therapy Code of Ethics indicates that we should be respectful of the cultural components of the recipients of our service. But beyond this point, a more recent and general concern has been voiced for the "sandwich generation," those caught between the obligation of caring for children and the obligation of caring for parents. Their needs must also be considered.

Who Are the Players?

The players are Mrs. Ciarrelli, her son, her daughter-in-law, their children, the occupational therapist, the home health agency, the family lawyer, neighbors, and the family physician. Are there any others?

What Other Information Is Needed?

How long has Mrs. Ciarrelli lived in her home? How long have her son and daughter-in-law lived with her? What is her relationship with her son and daughter-in-law, her grandchildren, and her neighbors? How old are her grandchildren? What time do they arrive home from school? Is there a senior center, a church, or a social group near her home? Do any of her friends participate in any of the activities at the senior center, church, or social group? Does a member of the clergy make home visits? Does Mrs. Ciarrelli have physical limitations? Is she mentally competent? What is her prognosis? Is she a candidate for some kind of home care, Meals on Wheels, or social services for elders? Are any other facts needed?

What Actions May Be Taken and What Are the Possible Consequences?

Mrs. Ciarrelli has the right to refuse service. If she does not want the occupational therapist to come into her home, she should not be required to receive this service. Although she is in the early stages of Alzheimer's disease and sometimes becomes confused, her refusal of occupational therapy does not necessarily make her mentally incompetent. A competent person is not always a rational person.

Competence may be tested by engaging the person in a process to determine how he or she relates to others and decides issues concerning participation in occupations that are meaningful to

Box 10-9 Summary

Competence may be tested by engaging the person in a process to determine how he or she relates to others and decides issues concerning participation in occupations that are meaningful to him or her, physical health, and finances.

her, physical health, and finances (Box 10-9). In essence, the ability to make a decision is a form of competence. Although we do not know whether Mrs. Ciarrelli has taken such a test, we do know that she made a decision that other family members did not like.

Is Mrs. Ciarrelli's refusal to see the therapist based on rational reasons? For some individuals of advanced years who are of a different cultural heritage from that of their visitors, the thought of a stranger coming into the home and telling them what to do is reason enough to refuse service. This may be Mrs. Ciarrelli's reason for not wanting the occupational therapist in her home. Her son and daughter-in-law do not want to neglect their mother; they want the best for her. How can all parties arrive at an understanding?

If Mrs. Ciarrelli is "incompetent," then her son is sanctioned to act in a paternalistic fashion as her guardian. He is seen as doing his duty when he decides what is good for his mother. Does Mrs. Ciarrelli understand that her behavior may result in this outcome? If so, does she prefer having her son make decisions for her rather than having outside help from a therapist? Perhaps overt paternalism is not the only solution.

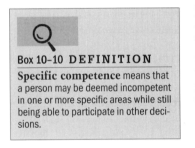

Box 10-10 DEFINITION

Specific competence means that a person may be deemed incompetent in one or more specific areas while still being able to participate in other decisions.

Box 10-11 *Summary*

A test for competence may assess a person's ability to offer a preference, to understand his or her own situation, and to reason through the consequences of a decision.

If Mrs. Ciarrelli's family chooses to have her tested for competence, they will have to pursue a legal determination. They may choose to use the concept of "specific incompetence," meaning that Mrs. Ciarrelli may be determined incompetent in one or more specific areas while still being able to participate in others of her own decisions (Box 10-10) (Beauchamp & Childress, 1994).

The decision to judge someone as incompetent is a moral as well as a medical and legal decision. Many tests are used to determine competence. Beauchamp and Childress (1994) offer a schema to express a range for evaluating competence. They cluster questions around the person's ability to offer a preference, to appreciate his or her situation, and to reason through the consequences of a decision (Box 10-11). Specific questions address whether the individual is unable to do the following:

- ▶ Give a preference
- ▶ Understand his or her situation or similar situations
- ▶ Understand information given to him or her
- ▶ Give rational reasons
- ▶ Give risk/benefit-related reasons
- ▶ Reach a reasonable decision based on the "reasonable person standard"

This schema could be used in Mrs. Ciarrelli's case to judge whether the family needs to take decision-making responsibilities away from her and whether she is competent, in this instance, to refuse occupational therapy.

Study Questions

1. Define the three elements of informed consent.

2. When is a situation justifiably considered an emergency that may require involuntary use of restraints or seclusion?

3. On what basis is a patient's competence to refuse or accept treatment judged?

4. As an occupational therapist, you expect to involve patients in treatment planning and to maintain confidentiality. Under what circumstances may these expectations be violated?

5. How can you avoid a breach of confidentiality or not respecting a patient's right to informed consent? How might you assess the patient's ability to weigh risks and benefits of treatment?

Informed Consent
in Research

CASE: Therapist Has Questions About Informed Consent

with commentaries by **Colin B. Gracey, DMin,**
and **Penny Kyler, MA, OTR, FAOTA**

Key Terms

Confidentiality   Privacy
Human subject (participant)   Privacy Rule

CASE: **Therapist Has Questions About**
Informed Consent

A large-scale research project is being conducted in a rehabilitation hospital with federal government funding. Sylvia Lopez, the occupational therapist, is asked by the principal investigator to submit data that she has gathered on her clients as part of her routine evaluation. Some of these clients have left the hospital, but Ms. Lopez has access to the evaluation data in their files.

Although the client participants gave consent to participate in the research study, they were unaware that their occupational therapy data would be used in the research. The principal investigator is not on the clinical staff of the hospital but claims, correctly, that it is not unusual for hospital-based researchers to request clinical data about participants that have been gathered for clinical purposes rather than for research purposes.

Who owns the data? Should specific consent be given by each participant for the occupational therapy data to be used in the study? Is the occupational therapist obligated to provide the data?

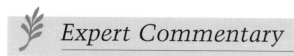

Expert Commentary

By Colin B. Gracey, DMin

This case provides an example of how an occupational therapy practitioner might become involved with human research. It raises questions about professional and healthcare personnel responsibilities when human research is undertaken or when human subject research becomes a component within or in addition to client care. Ms. Lopez needs to know the responsibilities that apply to clinical care and how these relate to those that apply to human subject research.

Involvement with those who conduct or participate in human research projects means involvement in the extensive and complex context of research to produce knowledge. Scientific, medical, business, government, institutional, and professional agencies seek to carry out human research in ways that add to scientific knowledge, protect human participants, maintain trust, and meet citizen expectations of the integrity, appropriate aims, means, and oversight of the enterprise of human research.

Research adds an additional interest to the traditional client–practitioner relationship and presents a potential for a conflict of interests. Under normal clinical circumstances, the clinician's goals presumably are purely coincident with those of the client. Under the construct of clinical research, an added goal, the goal of research, enters. In a hospital setting the difference research introduces is the difference between research with its attendant goals and clinical care with its goals. These goals are not mutually exclusive, but they are different. This difference may be conveyed in specific language. It is the difference between a "human subject" and a "patient" or "client" (Box 11-1). A "human subject" (now a referred to as participant) is a person who consents to participate in a research investigation. A "patient" or "client" is a person who contracts with a medical institution or professional for medical care.

Healthcare professionals may work with individuals who have consented to participate in research as such or with individuals who as clients have in addition consented to participate in research. In either

Box 11-1 *By the Law*

45 CFR 46 102(f) defines **human subject** (now referred to as **participant**) "Human subject means a living individual about whom an investigator (whether professional or student) conducting research obtains (1) data through intervention or interaction with the individual, or (2) identifiable private information."

case, healthcare professionals need to fulfill responsibilities that are associated with carrying out research involving humans. In this case scenario, when a client may also be a human participant, the occupational therapy practitioner needs to be clear about the primary nature of the contract for care that the client/participant has entered into with the medical professional or institution.

The Common Rule

The healthcare system in the United States has long been aware of the tension between the potential, significant benefits flowing from research and the primary and immediate obligations of care for human patients/participants. As a result, a body of work has been and is constantly being developed that addresses concerns and provides a framework within which research may proceed while protecting human participants. The statutory form of these developments at the federal level include the Code of Federal Regulations 45 CFR 46 (1991) (Common Rule) and the Code of the Food and Drug Administration (FDA) 21 CFR 50 and 56 (2000). The Common Rule (Box 11-2) applies strictly to research sponsored by the federal government, even though the National Bioethics Advisory Commission has recommended that Congress require all research (corporate-sponsored, academic, etc.) to be subject to the same rules. Also, federal statutory rules do not supersede statutory rules that may exist within state or local jurisdictions. In the case, the research project is being conducted in the rehabilitation hospital with federal government funding. Therefore, the stipulations of the Common Rule apply (or in case of a study involving drugs, the FDA rules apply).

> **Box 11-2**
>
> **Further Reading**
>
> For Common Rule requirements of an IRB with respect to privacy and confidentiality, see 45 CRF 46.111.

Institutional Resources to Educate, Help, and Guide

A medical or academic institution that does research sponsored by the federal government has a Human Research Office. The function of the Human Research Office includes establishing, supporting, and overseeing the following:

▶ Multiple Project Assurances with the Office of Human Research Protections (OHRP) within the Department of Health and Human Services (DHHS) and other assurances

▶ The work of an Institutional Review Board (IRB) (Box 11-3)

▶ An Institutional Compliance Division

▶ The administrative validation of agreements with research sponsors

▶ The formulation and promulgation of institutional policies and procedures with respect to research and the educational means

Box 11–3

Further Reading

For understanding the workings of an IRB, see "Institutional Review Board Management and Function," Robert Amdur and Elizabeth Bankert. (2002). Sudbury, MA: Jones and Bartlett Publishers.

and requirements expected of those within the institution to do or be involved with human research

The Human Research Office is the key local resource for all healthcare personnel who need to know about their responsibilities with regards to human research.

Regulations Relevant to the Case

In the case under consideration, Ms. Lopez will find that the Common Rule and existing policies having to do with human research directly affect and add to understandings that are operative within the Occupational Therapy Code of Ethics (2000a) and the Guidelines to the Occupational Therapy Code of Ethics (1998b).

In addition, she needs to be aware that by April 2003, compliance will be expected to a final version of "Standards for Privacy of Individually Identifiable Health Information" (the Privacy Rule) that was required by the Health Insurance Portability and Accountability Act (HIPAA) of 1996. This law will require written permission or authorization by clients/participants for their participation in a clinical trial or research and for use of their healthcare information in research. These permissions will need to be specifically stated and integrated into the research consent form. The consent form will need to state what medical information is to be used, how it may be used, by whom it will be used, and for how long the permission will be granted.

In the case under consideration, the consent form will need to state that permission is granted by the participant for the investigator to access their healthcare information, their medical records, and their occupational therapy evaluation data. The **Privacy Rule** is an attempt to provide additional privacy protections of healthcare information for clients and for those who participate in human research. This law will be enforced by the Office of Civil Rights within the DHHS and may impose liabilities on hospitals, healthcare providers, and research investigators in the form of fines and/or criminal sanctions. Compliance with the Common Rule, in contrast, is overseen by the OHRP within the DHHS. The OHRP can conduct audits, and in cases of noncompliance can issues warnings to investigators and institutions, suspend research, or, in more serious cases, temporarily suspend an institution's research programs.

Stakeholders

With human research, the stakeholders are many, the stakes are high indeed, but not more so than for the participant who deserves and requires carefully implemented procedures and protections. Stakeholders in the case scenario include, at least, the principal investigator and his or her department, the sponsor of the research, the hospital and hospital oversight groups, the IRB, the occupational therapy department, Sylvia Lopez, and her clients.

The Principal Investigator's Request

In the case under consideration, a principal investigator (PI), who is not a member of the clinical staff, asks Ms. Lopez for data she has gathered as part of her routine evaluation on her clients, including some who have left the hospital. Before answering this request, Ms. Lopez needs to know the status of the PI. Is the PI employed by the rehabilitation hospital? This might be required by the hospital for reasons of institutional liability. The clinical data of her clients cannot simply be released to a PI who is not a member of the clinical staff without possibly violating conditions of client privacy as well as confidentiality of a client's medical information (Boxes 11-4, 11-5).

Furthermore, the rehabilitation hospital IRB would have had to approve the research for it to be undertaken at the hospital. Ms. Lopez needs to know what is contained in the consent form of the approved research protocol. Depending on the provisions of the informed consent previously signed by the participants, there may be a need for reconsenting them for an explicit purpose, such as a new secondary use of data. Plus, there may possibly be a need for an interinstitutional contractual agreement denoting the methods of ensuring the confidentiality of the participants by the receiving organization if, for example, the PI were sharing data with investigators beyond the rehabilitation hospital.

Box 11-4

Further Reading

For Protection of Human Subjects (Informed Consent), see 21 CFR 50. For requirements of an IRB with respect of privacy and confidentiality, see 21 CFR 56.111.

Box 11-5 *Summary*

"**Privacy** can be defined in terms of having control over the extent, timing, and circumstances of sharing oneself (physically, behaviorally, or intellectually) with others. **Confidentiality** pertains to the treatment of information that an individual has disclosed in a relationship of trust and with the expectation that it will not be divulged to others in ways that are inconsistent with the understanding of the original disclosure without permission" (Office for Protection from Research Risks, OPRR Guidebook, 1993. Updated June 23, 2000).

Medical Data Access and Privacy/Confidentiality

A request for clinical data, therefore, raises issues for the occupational therapist in regard to her professional responsibilities concerning respecting the privacy of persons who are under or have been under her care as well as maintenance of the confidentiality of medical data that is part of or related to a person's medical record. The privacy issue generally rests on whether specific clients voluntarily gave their informed consent to participate in the research.

The issue of privacy often gets raised for potential research participants when they are "approached cold" by research investigators who seek their participation in research. Potential participants want to know how the investigator learned that they might be appropriate candidates to participate in a specific research project. Sometimes complaints are made to an IRB on this point because individuals believe their privacy with respect to their medical status has been violated. This situation is a problem both for investigators who seek to identify appropriate potential participants and for individuals who wonder how the investigators selected them.

A provision that mitigates but does not entirely resolve this problem is for investigators to inform primary care physicians or attending healthcare professionals of the nature of the research and ask these persons, who are familiar with their patients or clients, to ask them if they would be interested in learning about a research project. If the answer is "yes," then the investigator can be provided with the opportunity to approach the patient/client to explain the nature of the research and seek his or her participation.

This situation shows that with human research, privacy issues are involved from the beginning steps of recruitment, through the procedures of the proposed research, to the risks and benefits, and to the conditions of confidentiality that will be in place. These items need to be scrutinized and assessed by the IRB before its approval of a research project. The occupational therapy practitioner, therefore, needs to be knowledgeable about how privacy and confidentiality concerns are related to the consent form used in human research.

What Will Guide the Occupational Therapy Practitioner?

Clients who become participants in the research through appropriate consent procedures are considered to be human participants within an approved research project and, therefore, come under the privacy and confidentiality stipulations of the Common Rule. If these are the circumstances in the case scenario, Ms. Lopez can be guided about the release of the participant's clinical or evaluation data by the procedures and conditions stated in the research protocol. The conditions of confidentiality outlined in the consent form are particularly pertinent.

If the consent form mentions that the PI would require access to clinical data or to medical records as part of the research, and if the consent form outlined provisions to protect the confidentiality of the participant regarding the use of that data, then there is adequate authorization for Ms. Lopez to submit the evaluation data to the PI.

The IRB in giving its approval for the research would have considered issues such as the following:

▶ The use of identifiable data
▶ Plans to code or de-identify data
▶ The security of information that can link participant identification to codes
▶ Limitations on the use of data
▶ Destruction of identifiers and data upon completion of research
▶ Plans to publish research results in ways that will directly and indirectly protect confidentiality
▶ Whether there are plans to share research data or results with other researchers (this is allowed when data is anonymous)
▶ Who else beyond the PI, coinvestigators, and study staff might have access to the data, such as sponsors or persons authorized by law.

By being aware of the types of procedures needed to maintain confidentiality, Ms. Lopez can check that these issues have been addressed adequately in the confidentiality section of the consent form (Box 11-6).

Finally, the IRB would have considered whether appropriate accompanying documents, such as a medical records access form, was submitted with the protocol and consent form. This point would be of relevance for Ms. Lopez for her clients who have left the hospital.

Box 11-6 *Summary*

For online courses required of healthcare professionals involved in human participant research, see http://cme.nc.nih.gov or the Collaborative IRB Training Initiative (CITI) with case-based application of ethical principles and regulations, www.miami.edu/citireg.

Sometimes, consent forms are not clear about whether data beyond what is collected at the time of doing a research procedure will be gathered for follow-up or other research purposes, and yet this may be implied by statements in the confidentiality section of the consent form. For consent to be informed consent, however, procedures and provisions need to be clearly stated in understandable language. Also, research is sometimes approved that states in the protocol but only implies in the consent form that clinical data will be needed in the course of doing the research. The confidentiality section usually clarifies the situation when the procedure section is not explicit. When a research protocol comes before the IRB at the time of annual review (required by the Common Rule), clarifications and improvements to the consent form are often specified and must be made and implemented before the research can be approved for another year.

The point here is that if an occupational therapy practitioner has questions about the appropriateness of releasing clinical data or evaluation data to a PI, she can ask to see the research protocol and consent form and can assess whether the participants consented to having their medical data used in the research. She should also look to see if conditions are in place to protect the confidentiality of the data once it is handed over.

Dealing With a Perception Gap

Ms. Lopez would certainly raise questions about whether her clients consented to having their medical data released for research purposes if the clients, as stated in the case, conveyed that they were unaware that their occupational therapy data would be used in the research. In looking into the matter, Ms. Lopez might discover that her clients had technically consented to having their data used, although, as this case indicates, they were not aware of having done so. In this situation, before releasing any data, it would behoove her to explain this situation to each client involved. She needs to point out to them how they, in fact, did consent to their medical data being made available to the research investigator.

If upon this explanation her clients do not acknowledge this understanding for themselves, however, they must not be coerced into accepting that they had consented. They can withdraw from the research if they so choose and not have their data submitted to the PI. This provision for withdrawal is required by the Common Rule and will always be stated in the consent form.

With regard to clients who have left the hospital, unless there are other reasons to do so, these clients should not be contacted to explain the situation or to confirm whether they were aware of having given consent to have their medical data used. To accept that they in fact had given their consent to have the medical data used would be to avoid placing any additional burdens on them.

Ms. Lopez might also discuss with the PI the fact that a perception gap exists within the consent process of the research—in other words, what the participants technically consented to—as opposed to their understanding of what they thought they had consented to. This discussion could help the PI to consider rectifying the situation for future participants by submitting a clarifying amendment to the IRB and changing the consent form accordingly for future use.

When "No" is the Way to Go

If, on the other hand, Ms. Lopez discovered that the consent form had not stated or implied that clinical data would be needed or used for the research, she needs to inform the PI that she cannot supply the data requested and explain her reasons. These reasons, of course, have everything to do with her professional code of conduct to protect the privacy of clients and participants and to maintain the confidentiality of client medical data. She also has an obligation to follow hospital policies and commitments to clients regarding the confidentiality of their medical information.

An Educational Moment

This situation could be an educational moment for the PI and perhaps for the IRB. Such moments, as difficult as they may be, are actually in the service of improvements in the conduct of human research in institutional settings. Most PIs and IRBs will respond positively by making corrections or amendments to facilitate the research so it can go forward with additional participants.

Ordinarily, an IRB will not approve the reconsenting of participants or the supplemental consenting of participants who have participated in a research project to rectify a flawed protocol or consent form; however, appropriate corrections for the needs of the research can be incorporated by the PI into a revised protocol and consent form and can provide the basis for approval by the IRB for further research with additional or new participants.

Slippery Slope and Possible Consequences

Another option for Ms. Lopez might be for her to consider submitting the clients' evaluation data to be merely a matter of responding to the PI as a person in authority, or as a matter of simple cooperation. She might believe that supplying data is a relatively trivial matter given the importance of the research and simply decide to respond to the PI's request by providing the evaluation data.

This course, given the conditions stated in the case scenario, would represent a failure to fulfill her professional code of conduct responsibilities at several points as well as a failure to uphold hospital policy on confidentiality. Confidentiality of medical data means that disclosure requires permission by the client whose data it is. This lapse represents a serious violation of a client's rights and provides grounds for dismissal.

Furthermore, this option would not be of service to the PI. There is a real possibility that the IRB, upon receiving a progress report at the time of the annual review of the protocol and consent form, would identify discrepancies and take action to withhold approval until these issues were addressed. Also, if a participant or any other person aware of the situation were to file a complaint with the IRB, it could result in the need for the PI to file a protocol violation to the IRB, to account for what happened, and to explain what remedies would be undertaken. If a complaint were filed with the OHRP, this could also trigger an audit of the PI's research and result in sanctions being imposed. The OHRP also makes periodic audits of research sites, and these, too, take note of human research that may not be in compliance with stipulations as put forth by the Common Rule. So it is wise for all parties involved in human research to work together to get things right.

Reasons for Diligence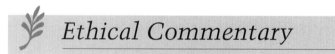

There are three additional reasons why utmost attention to proceeding with human research within the parameters of the Common Rule is important: (1) to protect research participants, (2) to not impede the benefits that research may provide through improved health care, and (3) to foster citizen trust and confidence in the system that carries out human research and relies on the citizenry for its continued funding and support.

Occupational therapy practitioners, along with many others, are crucial players in doing human research well. Human research involves various nuances that require informed attention, common sense, wise judgment, and accountability for decisions made.

Ethical Commentary

By Penny Kyler, MA, OTR, FAOTA

In considering this case, one should bear in mind that the profession is moving toward a master's degree at entry level. At that time, more occupational therapists will be expected to participate in research protocols. There is a learning curve and a level of competence that one should attain before conducting research and a level of knowledge needed to understand one's responsibilities as presented in this case scenario.

One resource for information is the OHRP. Before the OHRP can approve an Assurance, it must be satisfied that the institutional official, the Chair of the IRB, and the Human Protections Administrator at the institution understand the responsibilities involved in an institutional program of human participant protection. To do this, the OHRP has several Web-based tutorials for individuals to take, including several on informed consent (http://137.187.206.145/cbttng_ohrp/cbts/assurance/default.asp).

The occupational therapy Code of Ethics Principle 3 speaks to the concepts of informed consent. The Guidelines to the Code of Ethics further address the issues of data in Section 1.1 Honesty, where it is stated that practitioners must be honest in receiving and disseminating information; and in 2.9 regarding competence; and finally in 4.1 and 4.3, both of which indicate that the therapist should know the state and federal laws governing research. Occupational therapy educators are now embedding the basic components of research and the ethical obligations associated with research into their curricula.

Who Are the Players?

The players include Sylvia Lopez, the principal investigator, the funding agent, the clients or research participants, the occupational therapy department, and other clients. Are there others?

What Other Information Is Needed?

Other facts needed include: Who is Ms. Lopez's supervisor? What are the parameters of the research project? Will it last multiple years? How easy or difficult is it to get in touch with those clients/participants who have left the hospital? Will a lack of occupational therapy data make a difference to the research project? Might Ms. Lopez be invited to be a coauthor on any publication that results from the research? If so, what will the time commitment be, and is it likely to interfere with her work with clients?

What Actions May Be Taken and What Are the Possible Consequences?

Dr. Gracey has clearly indicated several actions that can be taken and the possible consequences; however, the reader should consider what would happen if a former client discovers data in a publication resulting from the research project that could be linked to him or her. Dr. Gracey notes that the former clients need not be contacted; however, Ms. Lopez has raised the question of whether these clients knowingly consented to their occupational therapy data being used in the project. If she feels sufficiently uncertain about this point, Ms. Lopez may wish to provide former clients with the name and phone number of the PI. Doing so would enable the clients to make an autonomous decision regarding participation in the study.

On a different point, if the principal investigator is asking for occupational therapy information to include in the study, one would assume that this information will need to be interpreted and put in a clinical context by Ms. Lopez, in which case she is now adding considerably to the study and might be invited to be a coauthor. It will be up to Ms. Lopez to weigh the advantages against obligations and time constraints regarding participation as a coauthor in the study. Will participating in the project affect client care? Would there be constraints based on the size of her caseload? It is certainly possible and desirable for occupational therapy practitioners to participate in both clinical work and research at the same time. In fact, occupational therapists are usually open to inquiry and enjoy problem solving, both of which are employed in research as well as in clinical practice. Ms. Lopez is faced with a problem when making the decision to participate in the research study or not; however, this particular problem is ethically solvable and is therefore not strictly speaking a dilemma.

Editor's note: The fact that the two experts have differing opinions about whether to notify the former clients probably indicates that Ms. Lopez is faced with an ethical dilemma on that particular point.

Study Questions

1. Where is the potential conflict of interest when a client is also a research participant?
2. What is the responsibility of participants of a health professional conducting research?
3. When does the Common Rule apply, and what is the role of the Human Research Office?
4. What is the Privacy Rule, and how does it affect occupational therapy practice and research?
5. How do privacy and confidentiality differ? How are these rights protected in human participant research and through the Occupational Therapy Code of Ethics?

Contracts and Referrals to Private Practice

CASE: Absence of a Written Contract

with commentaries by **Milton Schwartzberg, JD,** *and* **Penny Kyler MA, OTR, FAOTA**

Key Terms

Apparent authority	Legal capacity
Contractual obligation	Quasi-contracts
Express contract	Reasonable payment
Implied contract	Utilitarianism

CASE: Absence of a Written Contract

Sue has cerebral palsy and uses a wheelchair. She has been working at a sheltered workshop for several months and has just acquired a competitive job; however, she needs an adapted switch to do the job successfully. The engineer at the workshop calls a friend, an occupational therapist, for help with the adaptive switch.

The occupational therapist has taken the switch home to work on it and has put in considerable time, effort, creative expertise, and money for supplies. When it is complete, the occupational therapist sends the engineer a bill for his labor and supplies; however, the engineer claims that she thought the therapist was doing this out of consideration for the client and says there is no money to pay for such a service.

The occupational therapist is in a dilemma. He has no written agreement with the engineer or with the workshop or with Sue but believes he should be paid for his work and expertise. Sue cannot start work until she has the switch. Should the occupational therapist give Sue the switch and continue negotiating with the engineer? Should he withhold the switch until he is paid—either by the engineer, the workshop, or Sue?

Introduction and Update

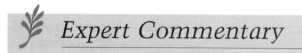

Expert Commentary

By Milton Schwartzberg, JD

Unlike the chapter dealing with the Family Educational Rights and Privacy Act (FERPA) statute and issues of privacy (Chapter 2), the law of contracts is relatively static. We examine how a statutory regulation enacted by Congress can have far-reaching implications in higher education. The dynamic component involving the case law interpretation of this statute makes its scope ever changing. Accordingly, the scenario described in the FERPA chapter can be subject to repeated modification to conform with changes in the application of the statute based on findings made in cases that interpret this law even further.

In contrast, the fundamentals of a contract and its enforceability have been a cornerstone of U.S. civil law for many years. Much of U.S. commerce would not be possible without the stability this body of law provides. Even an occupational therapy practitioner in a transaction involving relatively small amounts of financial remuneration can benefit from the same legal principles that the largest corporations in the United States rely on every day. This proven reliability and predictability make any wholesale revision of the first edition text unnecessary. The definitions, analysis, and advice given at that time are equally valid today.

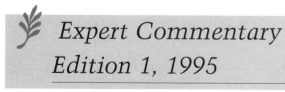

Expert Commentary
Edition 1, 1995

By Milton Schwartzberg, JD

In many years of practicing law, the questions and ambiguities raised in this scenario have regularly repeated themselves. In representing a diverse cross-section of business clients, these same issues were the common source of much client consternation.

Over the last 20 years, I have seen the profession of occupational therapy grow and achieve an ever-expanding prominence in the health sciences field. It is inevitable that this success and recognition will be accompanied by an ever-increasing encroachment of the business world. Occupational therapy practitioners will be increasingly faced with situations in which their expectations and goals will be merged with legal, financial, and business considerations.

My objective is to enable the reader to obtain a fundamental understanding of the law of contracts; of how this law can be a friend, not a foe, as well as its practical application for the practitioner.

The subject scenario needs clarity and a clear delineation of intent among the three parties; the forces of ambiguity are at the root of the dilemma. In examining the options, one is struck by the fact that all of the parties are well-intentioned. Unfortunately, any finding or ruling would have a negative impact on one or more of the participants as the elusive quality of justice is sought.

In examining the situation, what is *not* said is as important as what is said. For example, possible first questions to ask either the occupational therapist or the engineer include: "What did each of you say?" "What was your understanding at the conclusion of your discussion and before you commenced work?"

The fact pattern is cleverly crafted to enable an advocate for any of the parties to make a credible argument. Before delving into a discussion of the rights of the individuals involved, a brief overview of contract law is appropriate.

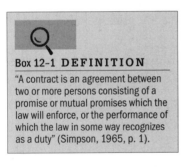

Box 12-1 DEFINITION

"A contract is an agreement between two or more persons consisting of a promise or mutual promises which the law will enforce, or the performance of which the law in some way recognizes as a duty" (Simpson, 1965, p. 1).

Contracts and Contract Law

Formally defined, "a contract is an agreement between two or more persons consisting of a promise or mutual promises which the law will enforce, or the performance of which the law in some way recognizes as a duty" (Simpson, 1965, p. 1) (Box 12-1).

The less formal definition is that a contract is "a promise or set of promises which the law will enforce" (Simpson, 1965, p. 1). The promise or promises may be either verbal or written. Although verbal contracts are enforceable, practical considerations strongly favor written contracts. By reducing these promises to writing, the understanding and obligations of the participants are defined and presumably agreed upon (Box 12-2).

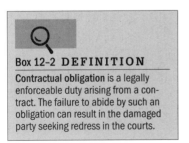

Box 12-2 DEFINITION

Contractual obligation is a legally enforceable duty arising from a contract. The failure to abide by such an obligation can result in the damaged party seeking redress in the courts.

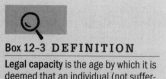

Box 12-3 DEFINITION

Legal capacity is the age by which it is deemed that an individual (not suffering from severe mental or emotional impairment) can enter into binding contracts and other acts. This is frequently referred to as the "age of majority." In most jurisdictions in the United States this age is 18 years.

Verbal agreements, on the other hand, rely on the memory and integrity of the participants. Unfortunately, self-interest may color a participant's memory. It is rare that two parties to a verbal contract agree completely on its contents after it has been formed. The passage of time tends to promote further differences in these recollections.

Following are the four elements essential to the formation of a contract:

1. The participants are (two or more) persons over the age of majority (18 in most jurisdictions), being of sound mind. Entities such as corporations, partnerships, and trusts may also enter into a contract. A person or entity capable of entering into a contract is said to have the *legal capacity* to do so (Box 12-3).
2. These parties must agree to the terms, conditions, and objectives of the contract. This is known as *mutual assent.*
3. Something of value must be exchanged between the parties. This is referred to as *legal consideration* or simply consideration.
4. The subject matter or objective of the contract must be legal. For example, an agreement to commit a crime would not be considered a contract and, therefore, is unenforceable. Because human conduct rarely conforms to the strict requirements that the law sets down, the wisdom of English common law (which is inherited) has proven to be most flexible. Situations present themselves (such as the scenario in this chapter) that defy strict definition within the conventional elements of a contract. Fortunately, the law of contracts has evolved to accommodate these circumstances.

True contracts are those in which obligation arises from actual agreement and intent of the parties to promise. If the agreement or mutual assent is manifested in words, oral or written, the contract is said to be "express." On the other hand, where the mutual undertaking of the parties is inferred from conduct alone, without spoken or written words, the contract is said to be "implied in fact." In either case, a real agreement is manifested (Simpson, 1965, p. 5).

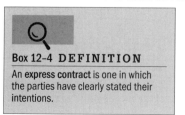

Box 12-4 DEFINITION

An **express contract** is one in which the parties have clearly stated their intentions.

Simply put, an *express contract* is one in which the parties have clearly stated their intentions (Box 12-4). In an *implied contract*, the conduct of the parties is of paramount importance in

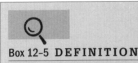

Box 12-5 DEFINITION

An **implied contract** (or implied-in-fact contract) is one in which the conduct of the parties is of paramount importance in determining whether a contract exists.

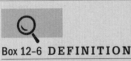

Box 12-6 DEFINITION

Quasi-contracts (or implied-in-law contracts) are contracts in which the parties fail to conform to contractual prerequisites, but justice requires an obligation of payment. These are not considered legal contracts but rather situations in which the absence of payment or compensation would be manifestly unjust. Only a court of law can make such a determination based on the merits of each case.

determining whether a contract exists (Box 12-5). Note that the legal obligations of the parties to either an express or implied contract are no different because each contract is legally enforceable.

In addition, there are situations in which the parties fail to conform to contractual prerequisites, but justice requires an obligation of payment. These are known as contracts "implied in law" or "quasi-contracts" (Box 12-6). Note that these are not considered legal contracts but rather situations in which the absence of payment or compensation would be manifestly unjust. Only a court of law could make such a determination based on the merits of each case.

Conduct Vis-à-vis Elements of a Contract

To better understand the rights and duties of the occupational therapist, the engineer, and Sue, their respective conduct vis-à-vis the fundamental elements of a contract must be discussed.

First, although ages are not mentioned, it appears that all parties are above the age of majority. It further appears that no mental impairment affects the ability of any of the parties to enter into a contract. It appears then that all parties have the legal capacity to enter into the contract.

In many ambiguous contractual situations, determining mutual assent is considerably more difficult. In most circumstances, mutual assent manifests itself by an offer made by one party and acceptance by the other party. This offer and acceptance are at face value. Moreover, the validity of mutual assent is not affected if either party has a hidden agenda or ulterior motive in making the offer, or accepting it. The law relies on the apparent sincerity of the offer and acceptance in determining whether mutual assent exists.

In other words, an offer is any communication made to a party who, by agreeing to its terms, will be contractually bound. Offers, if not rejected outright, may be withdrawn. They may also expire by their own terms or by the expiration of a reasonable amount of time. Offers may also be extinguished by the party receiving the offer (offeree), who may make another proposal known as a *counteroffer*.

Naturally, if the offering party becomes incapacitated in the interim or if the offer subsequently becomes illegal, it is no longer valid. These questions now present themselves: Was a valid offer made here? By and to whom? The engineer at the workshop calls her friend, an occupational therapist. Unfortunately, none of their conversation is revealed; however, as a result of their communication, the occupational therapist commences work on the adaptive device.

Certain inferences may be made as a result of this conduct. Clearly, at least one party (the occupational therapist) had taken the communication with the engineer to be an offer. He subsequently accepted this perceived offer by purchasing materials and building the switch. From his conduct, he appears to have intended consummating the contract by fully complying with what he believed to be an offer.

The next issue that arises is this: If the engineer actually communicated an offer to the occupational therapist, on whose behalf was this offer made? The engineer's? The sheltered workshop's? Sue's? To answer this question, an area of the law closely related to contracts known as agency must be explored. Among other things, this area of law deals with questions and issues arising from situations in which one person or entity acts on behalf of another. Questions often arise about whether a substitute person or agent can legally enter into a contract on someone else's behalf.

Most people are familiar with their local insurance agent, who usually represents several insurance companies. He or she is able to bind any of these companies into a contract of insurance by accepting the payment of a premium by a customer, so this agency situation is clear; however, is the engineer acting on anyone's behalf?

This question can be readily answered by examining the concept in agency law known as apparent authority (Box 12-7). Essentially, this doctrine means that when a person or entity allows another to appear to have the authority to act on his or her behalf, this person can be contractually bound. The doctrine's purpose is not to impede commerce by prospective customers having to prove or confirm that a company representative really did have the authority to act on the company's behalf. If the company permitted an individual to be on its premises and appear to act on its behalf, it could be held responsible if this individual entered into a contract. This would apply even if the individual was specifically told not to do so. The interests of the unsuspecting public were held to be higher than the company that willingly or unwillingly allowed this situation to exist.

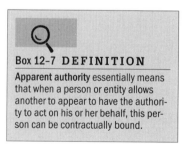

Box 12-7 DEFINITION

Apparent authority essentially means that when a person or entity allows another to appear to have the authority to act on his or her behalf, this person can be contractually bound.

Based on the scenario, it appears as if the engineer had the apparent authority to bind her employer (the sheltered workshop) into a contract with the occupational therapist. The specifics or job duties of the engineer are not stated. The workshop could argue that the engineer had no permission to contact suppliers to the workshop. In all likelihood, other employees would typically order supplies and the production of adaptive devices on behalf of the sheltered workshop.

The workshop could also argue that because the occupational therapist and engineer were friends, he knew that she did not and could not order these devices on the sheltered workshop's behalf. Because these arguments are all hypothetical, one can only go with the preponderance of evidence here. Even though the occupational therapist and engineer are friends, I believe that there is sufficient apparent authority to at least hold the sheltered workshop to have made an offer to the occupational therapist.

The sheltered workshop could make a credible argument that the engineer was an agent acting on behalf of Sue, or acting on her own. Because Sue was not working at the workshop when these communications took place, the workshop's position becomes even more substantial.

Before an ultimate decision and attempt to answer the questions posed at the conclusion of the scenario can be made, the law of contracts must be further examined.

It appears as if the engineer made an offer; however, was there a valid acceptance of this offer? This topic was briefly touched on earlier during the discussion of the fact that the occupational therapist produced the adaptive device in response to the apparent request of the engineer.

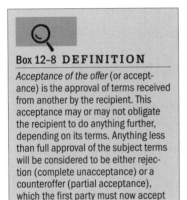

Box 12-8 DEFINITION

Acceptance of the offer (or acceptance) is the approval of terms received from another by the recipient. This acceptance may or may not obligate the recipient to do anything further, depending on its terms. Anything less than full approval of the subject terms will be considered to be either rejection (complete unacceptance) or a counteroffer (partial acceptance), which the first party must now accept or reject.

To be valid, the acceptance of the offer (1) must be made by the person or entity to whom the offer is communicated; (2) must conform to the specifics of the offer; and (3) must be made to the offering party (Box 12-8).

It appears clear under these circumstances that the offer made was not rejected. Rejection occurs not only by responding negatively to an offer, but also by varying the terms of the offer. When this happens, in effect, the response is a new offer that the original offering party can either accept or reject.

Once again, because the communication between the engineer and the occupational therapist was not stated, inferences must be made based on their conduct. The occupational therapist has apparently taken home the switch "to work on it." Presumably, this was done with the knowledge and consent of the engineer. Therefore, we can make several assumptions in attempting to determine whether the engineer's offer was accepted by the occupational therapist. Because these two parties were the only persons involved in the communication, it is safe to infer that the occupational therapist made the acceptance of the offer on his own. He evidently knew what adaptations the engineer desired and actually performed them.

The problems arise around the question of payment and the apparent failure of the parties to discuss this issue. The respective claims of the participants in this scenario must now be evaluated. In attempting to reach an equitable solution, a court of law often looks to custom, usage, and practice in a given field as well as to what a reasonable and prudent person would expect and how he or she would behave. All of these factors, as well as personal experience and common sense (if a jury is involved), are components of the evaluative processes that eventually lead to a legal finding.

In most jurisdictions, juries sit only on the more serious criminal cases as well as on civil cases involving larger amounts of damages. If the scenario presented were ever before a court, the likelihood is that the damages involved would not justify a jury trial; however, a court would seek testimony in determining whether customary practices in the field of occupational therapy might occasionally include gratuitously constructing adaptive equipment for persons with disabilities.

If this were a typical practice or charitable gesture, then the engineer's offer takes on a new meaning. The engineer may then maintain that she reasonably expected her occupational therapist friend to perform these services at no charge. Furthermore, she could also claim that her friend was acting within the bounds of custom in the field, if, in fact, such a custom does exist.

Conversely, if this is not a customary method of providing these types of services, then the argument for reasonable payment to the occupational therapist becomes much more viable (Box 12-9). His position would be credible if he were to maintain that any reasonable person would be aware that his performance of the requested services would entail the purchase of supplies as well as the expenditure of skilled labor.

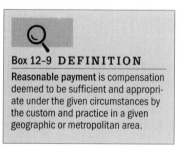

Box 12-9 DEFINITION

Reasonable payment is compensation deemed to be sufficient and appropriate under the given circumstances by the custom and practice in a given geographic or metropolitan area.

Under these circumstances, I believe that a reasonable person would conclude that the occupational therapist would be entitled to remuneration for his efforts. Furthermore, he also becomes the unintended recipient of a primer in contracts law. His experience has most certainly taught him that vagueness and ambiguity are costly. These costs are not strictly monetary.

In the situation posed, the awkwardness and embarrassment that all parties must have experienced was most unpleasant. The business relationship among them suffered as well. Good intentions, although in abundance here, were not enough to avoid a good deal of unpleasantness.

Conclusions

Because the precise conversations between the engineer and the occupational therapist are not stated, it would be difficult to assume that there was an express contract. The conduct of the parties must be examined in an attempt to make a determination.

Accordingly, the respective actions of the parties appear to satisfy the requirements of an "implied-in-fact" contract. As previously stated, this type of contract is equally as valid as an express contract. Its inequality is not in its validity, but rather in the proving of its existence.

At the very least, a court of law would award payment to the occupational therapist on the theory of a quasi-contract or a contract "implied-in-law." Clearly, it would be unjust for the occupational therapist not to be compensated for his labor and material expenditures under these circumstances.

I also believe that the sheltered workshop would also likely be responsible for payment. This is based on the apparent authority that they permitted to exist in this situation. I would advise the occupational therapist to give the switch to the engineer or another authorized person at the sheltered workshop along with an itemized bill for labor and materials. I would further advise him to write a letter addressed to the workshop, which would be sent with the bill. The letter should review the pertinent events. The fact that the work was performed and the materials were purchased pursuant to a request for these services and assistance made by the engineer, a workshop employee, should be particularly emphasized. Unless there was a clear agreement to the contrary, the occupational therapist is justified in receiving reasonable compensation and reimbursement for materials purchased.

I would advise the occupational therapist to present the workshop with the switch at the time that the bill is sent. Because the workshop appears to be obligated to pay for the switch, they are entitled to possess it as well.

The occupational therapist should also inform Sue that he has given the switch to the workshop and that she should contact the workshop to arrange to pick up the device. All of the participants in this scenario probably have received a poignant, albeit unsolicited, lesson in the law of contracts and agency. Naturally, this costly lesson could have been avoided if the parties had been more direct with each other.

Clarity of Contract

As stated earlier, the practice of occupational therapy has been more involved than ever with the business world. Its ever-increasing prominence will undoubtedly make business considerations an everyday fact of life in the profession.

Fundamental advice that I give to business clients is to strive for clarity in all of their dealings. This point encompasses employee interactions as well as all types of transactions with other businesses. Ambiguity is your enemy; it breeds and fosters problems. In addition, well-intentioned and honorable persons striving to do "the right thing" can still run into serious problems when clarity is absent.

Promoting clarity is not synonymous with written contracts containing fine print and legalese. In the scenario in this chapter, a simple letter of understanding drafted and initialed by the participants would have been sufficient. If you find yourself in the position of writing such a letter or memo, keeping it simple works best for everyone. Essentially you are memorializing what is expected of you and the other parties. Your memo should basically be divided between the expectations that you have and those of the other party or parties. Simple transactions such as the scenario presented here do not require anything more than a brief letter or memo reiterating the offer, acceptance, and terms (including payment and reimbursement) of the transaction. It is not necessary to have a lawyer on standby. It is helpful to consult an attorney for questions or concerns, but it is not necessary for the more simple interactions encountered in most occupational therapy settings.

When an occupational therapy practice is involved in repeated transactions of a particular nature, such as procuring or producing adaptive devices, consulting an attorney is suggested as being good practice and being cost effective. An attorney would be able to draft a sample form contract or provide a checklist for use by the occupational therapy practitioner in drafting future memoranda. Otherwise, a good general rule to follow would be to thoroughly discuss a proposed transaction with the other party, then summarize in writing what is expected of each party. When the summary is agreeable to all, the firm foundation of a contract is established. A formal contract may be drafted, but this step may not be necessary if the contractual components previously discussed have been incorporated into the summary. A signature or initialing of the agreement signifies that the parties wish to be bound by the terms contained therein.

Make the summary/agreement as simple as possible. Unnecessary complexity defeats the objective of promoting clarity. Complexity also promotes ambiguity. If an attempt to reduce an understanding, agreement, or transaction to writing cannot avoid being complex, it is time to consult an attorney. In most instances, however, clarity of purpose and intent can be fully performed by the occupational therapy practitioner who is working in a private practice setting.

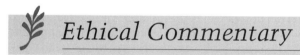

Ethical Commentary

By Penny Kyler, MA, OTR, FAOTA

The legal solution to the dilemma raised in the case example, "Absence of a Written Contract," is clear. A contract would have allowed all parties to function with complete understanding. The customary, prevailing, and reasonable charge method for determining charges for services is an accepted approach in healthcare practice and in business; however, practitioners are also concerned with the ethical issues raised by the dilemma in the case. The Guidelines to the Occupational Therapy Code of Ethics (AOTA, 1998b) indicate that it is acceptable and right to participate in bartering and pro bono work. Guideline 9: Payment for Services, notes that although bartering and pro bono work is not a common occurrence in the profession, it is still done. These options may be applicable when it is culturally appropriate and within the guidelines of the employer. These concepts open up other options for the players in this case.

Who Are the Players?

Sue, the engineer, the workshop staff, the workshop administration, the other clients, and the occupational therapist are the players. Are there other players?

What Other Information Is Needed?

Does the engineer request help with devices for many of her clients? Should she have been able to modify the switch without outside help? Does the occupational therapist commonly consult on making such devices? If so, what types of arrangements for pay has he made in the past? Have the parties entered into other agreements? Is there another job that Sue can do at her new place of employment until the disagreement is settled? Is any other information needed?

What Actions May Be Taken and What Are the Possible Consequences?

Occupational therapy practitioners have a duty to provide service to clients, but the decision to provide such service should not be predicated solely on payment. Ethical healthcare practitioners are guided by the fundamental belief in the worth of their clients. This belief is based on social responsibility, as stated in the AOTA Code of Ethics (AOTA, 2000a) and in the Standards of Practice (AOTA, 1998a). An ethical occupational therapy practitioner treats clients and delivers services not simply because of a contractual agreement, but because of a social responsibility to do so. The professional philosophy of engagement in meaningful occupations and activities helps practitioners focus on the betterment of those receiving their services. Designing or fabricating an adaptive device is one concrete way of helping a person to be a productive worker in society.

This case could be resolved using a utilitarian ethical approach (Box 12-10). The concept of utilitarianism is that moral right or wrong is judged by the nature of the consequences following the action for everyone involved (Beauchamp & Childress, 1994). In this case, everyone

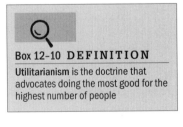

Box 12-10 DEFINITION

Utilitarianism is the doctrine that advocates doing the most good for the highest number of people

includes Sue, the engineer, the occupational therapist, the sheltered workshop, and the future employer.

From a utilitarian viewpoint, one good consequence would result if the therapist were to enter into a contractual arrangement with Sue, whereby she could pay for the device on an installment plan after she has been working for several weeks. Sue would benefit because she would be able to self-actualize and fulfill her role to work; the occupational therapist would benefit because he would be paid for his services; and the future employer would benefit by gaining a needed employee.

Another approach would be for Sue to be given the device at the same time as a bill for services is submitted to the workshop; this would allow Sue to be gainfully employed. Limiting her access to employment may be cause for a lawsuit, and it may also place undue hardship on Sue in regards to paying her bills and attending to other daily tasks. Not being employed while waiting for the assistive device may also trigger some self-doubts within Sue and lead to depression.

Occupational therapy practitioners have a *prima facie* duty of nonmaleficence (Box 12-11). Ross (1988) identifies nonmaleficence as a fundamental duty that instructs practitioners not to do anything that would injure another (Box 12-12). *Prima facie* duties occur when all other things are equal; however, a greater moral rule could override these duties. A person faced with a *prima facie* duty of nonmaleficence cannot ignore that duty simply because he or she would be inconvenienced as an individual. The occupational therapist in the scenario would not have lived up to his duty of nonmaleficence if he withheld the device from Sue because he would be depriving her of her ability to work. This is the case, even though he is being considerably inconvenienced by not being paid for his work.

> **Box 12-11 *Summary***
>
> *Prima facie* literally means at first sight or before closer inspection. A *prima facie* duty is an obligation that by its very nature has precedence over others. An example of this is the duty of a parent to care for a child.

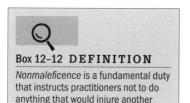

> **Box 12-12 DEFINITION**
>
> *Nonmaleficence* is a fundamental duty that instructs practitioners not to do anything that would injure another (Ross, 1988)

In occupational therapy, the duty of nonmaleficence is covered under Principle 2 (nonmaleficence) of the Code of Ethics (AOTA, 2000a). The principle instructs therapists to take all reasonable precautions to avoid harm to the recipient of services or detriment to the recipient's property. In addition, Principle 1.B allows therapists to enter into agreements with clients and states that a therapist "shall establish fees, based on cost analysis, that are commensurate with services rendered." This principle seems to indicate that the therapist in the case scenario was justified in expecting to be paid a fair price for his work, but that he should have entered into an agreement concerning payment before he started work on the device.

Times have changed, and more and more individuals with disabilities will seek information and devices directly from Web-based resources. Providing good services at no cost or bartering may be one of the best ways for occupational therapy practitioners to demonstrate the wealth of their skills and the good outcomes that may arise from an interaction with the profession. Sometimes doing a good deed is worth more in the long run than seeking the short-term goal of immediate remuneration.

Study Questions

1. Define the term *contract* and give the advantages of a written versus a verbal contract.

2. What are four essential elements in the formation of a contract?

3. What is *apparent authority*, and are there circumstances under which an occupational therapist may be free from such a contractual obligation?

4. What types of ethical dilemmas can the occupational therapy practitioner avoid by drafting written contracts?

5. When reimbursement is withheld or unavailable, what is the ultimate authority over whether an occupational therapy practitioner is ethically or legally bound to deliver a service? In this instance, are professional, legal, and ethical obligations the same?

The Whistleblower

CASE: The Whistleblower

With commentary by **Thomas G. Gutheil, MD,**
and **Penny Kyler, MA, OTR, FAOTA**

Key Terms

Disinterested party
Mandated reporter
Mediation

Protections
Retaliation
Whistleblower

CASE: The Whistleblower

Ching Mae Wong has been an occupational therapist for more than 25 years. She is currently a member of an interdisciplinary team making home visits to elders living in the community. The team does outreach in a predominantly suburban area with single-dwelling homes and small apartment buildings. Most residents in the community are working, and the few elderly people are most often parents needing care.

Ms. Wong has completed her initial assessment of Mr. Donabedian, an 80-year-old retired teacher living with his youngest daughter and her young child. On repeated occasions she has noticed bruises on her client's upper extremities. When Ms. Wong has inquired, both father and daughter change the subject or minimize the injuries. One morning she finds Mr. Donabedian alone in the apartment dazed and noncommunicative. The daughter does not answer her phone at work upon several attempts by the therapist.

Ms. Wong's supervisor ignores her concerns about the potential of abuse. For several weeks she has attempted to discuss the matter and he has been abrupt while reminding her of his status in the community as a school committee member. Without discussion, he has cut back her hours. The supervisor repeatedly smells of alcohol, rambles at meetings, and is explosive. Ms. Wong is fearful for her job and is tempted not to report the possibility of abuse to the health authorities.

What issues are raised concerning whistleblowing and retribution for following a professional duty to report abuse?

The Role of the Whistleblower

The whistleblower occupies a special place in organized systems such as corporations, institutions, businesses, and bureaucracies; whistleblowers are both precious and necessary (Box 13-1). The whistleblower boldly opposes the forces of inertia, entrenched policy, group solidarity that circles the wagons, dominance by an institutional power elite, and frank fear of reprisals to call attention to wrongs and abuses that might otherwise be swamped and silenced by the aforementioned forces. Whistleblowers commonly expose both abuse of persons and abuse of the system itself (Box 13-2). Although mature systems and persons welcome constructive feedback and information about problems to improve operations, less mature, narcissistically vulnerable, marginally competent decision makers or those who are highly identified for self-image with the system (like the supervisor here, puffed with his status as school committee member) often perceive presented opportunities for change or abuse prevention as a threat to the status quo and may resist, rebuff, or retaliate against such feedback on the basis that it rocks the boat.

The whistleblower often emerges from lower ranks, closer to the action, partly because decision makers higher in the system may be too remote from the action even to be aware of abuses (Box 13-3). In the case example, for instance, the whistleblower is the one who actually goes out to the clients to deliver services and observes the problems first hand.

Unfortunately, whistleblowing poses some problems in addition to its benefits. Like many valued processes, it can be corrupted by misuse to manipulate the system. One such event is **retaliation** from below for slights or injuries received from above. For example, the system in which Ms. Wong functions might respond to her

---

Box 13-1 *Summary*

The **whistleblower** occupies a special place in organized systems; whistleblowers are both precious and necessary.

Box 13-2 *Summary*

Whistleblowers commonly expose both abuse of persons and abuse of the system itself.

Box 13-3 *Summary*

Whistleblowers often emerge from the lower ranks, close to the action.

Box 13-4 *Summary*

The most effective whistleblowing is accomplished by the most **disinterested parties**—those with the least to gain and the least to lose.

complaint as though she were merely retaliating against her superiors for their having cut back her hours. One clear implication of this example is that the most effective whistleblowing is accomplished by the most disinterested parties (Box 13-4). In addition to the client's problems, the supervisor appears to be impaired by substance abuse; that situation, too, may be the subject of whistleblowing in some cases.

Protections

Does the whistleblower enjoy any protections against inappropriate retaliations? Several jurisdictions and some abuse statutes provide immunities for whistleblowers under many circumstances and protection

Box 13-5 *By the Law*

Most statutes that mandate reporting for various forms of abuse incorporate **protections** to encourage that reporting.

against retaliation. Most statutes that mandate reporting for various forms of abuse incorporate protections to encourage that reporting (Box 13-5).

In fact, the law provides both a carrot and a stick, so to speak. The whistleblower/ **mandated reporter** receives protection from a claim of breach of confidentiality or privilege as might otherwise be brought and protection from civil liability (e.g., libel). On the stick side, certain penalties accrue for *failure* to report those forms of abuse in the statute.

For example, the Massachusetts child abuse statute is typical of this format. It designates as mandated reporter all forms of caretaker, thus:

> Any physician, medical intern, hospital personnel engaged in the examination, care or treatment of persons, medical examiner, psychologist, emergency medical technician, dentist, nurse, chiropractor, podiatrist, osteopath, public or private school teacher, educational administrator, guidance or family counselor, day care worker or any person paid to care for or work with a child in any public or private facility or home or program funded by the Commonwealth. . . . Any of these who has reasonable cause to believe that a child under the age of eighteen years is suffering physical or emotional injury . . . must report same.
>
> (Massachusetts General Laws, c.119, section 51a)

The same statute states the immunity:

> No person so required to report shall be liable in any civil or criminal action by reason of such report. No other person making such report shall be liable in any civil or criminal action by reason of such report if it was made in good faith.
>
> (Massachusetts General Laws, c.119, section 51a)

Subsequent paragraphs prohibit retaliation and/or discrimination by employers. In the case example, Mr. Donabedian might qualify for statutes (with similar explicit protections) mandating reporting of either elder abuse or abuse of the mentally ill, depending on jurisdiction.

Beyond these legal requirements are ethical mandates that accompany professional status. These mandates might include the requirement of always acting in the client's interests and attempting to prevent harms. These mandates may require that Ms. Wong take action even in the face of an explicit or implied threat of retaliation, knowing that she is likely to receive statutory protection for doing so (and possible penalties for not doing so).

Alternatives to whistleblowing may also be relevant. Ms. Wong may have access to and be expected to employ established institutional grievance procedures to bring a potential problem issue to the attention of the system. In this instance, the institution is the home health agency by which she is employed.

Finally, institutional policy may provide both protections and confidentiality rules that, regrettably, are often only variably enforced and followed. The dilemma here is that a facility in which possible abuse has occurred may resist, deny, or otherwise hinder the reporting: the on-site whistleblower, after all, is blowing the whistle on himself or herself, in effect, as well as the institution (Box 13-6). Institutions usually provide in their policies and procedures information or requirements governing the path that such reporting should take (e.g., the employee may be instructed to notify a supervisor, unit head, or other person). Note also that an institution has the right to perform its own investigation, exploration, or inquiry before deciding to go outside the facility to involve other agencies.

> **Box 13-6 *Summary***
>
> Institutional policy may provide both protections and confidentiality rules that, regrettably, may not be followed because it is often the institution itself in which the possible abuse has occurred.

Retaliations

In the case example, a possible retaliation has occurred in the form of a cutback on Ms. Wong's hours after she reported the problem. Other possible but unfortunately not uncommon forms of retaliation include firing, transfer, ostracism, or forms of blackening the reputation of the whistleblower through negative job references, career assassinations, or even deliberate rumor spreading.

Support Strategies

The whistleblower can follow some practices that may militate in favor of greater success and more safety. First among these is the paper trail: a

Box 13-7 *Summary*

The whistleblower should maintain meticulous documentation of all details in the scenario.

Box 13-8 *Summary*

A second person who acts as witness and consultant can be invaluable in decreasing isolation and risk for the potential whistleblower.

Box 13-9 *Summary*

Mediation can often be helpful between the whistleblower and his or her supervisor.

practice of meticulous documentation of all details in the situation. In the case example, this method would include the observations of the physical signs of possible abuse, the calls made and not answered, and the conversations where the parties avoided the topic (Box 13-7).

Next in importance are the functions of witness and consultant; under some circumstances these could be the same person. A second observer of the clinical data and a peer who might help in gaining perspective on the situation and confirming the observations may be invaluable in decreasing the isolation and solitary risk for the potential whistleblower (Box 13-8).

The tension between Ms. Wong and her supervisor might also be mitigated by the use of mediation approaches; these would not be limited to use of professional mediators but might be accomplished by individuals in the system itself, be they peers or senior staff (Box 13-9). Which is better—in-house mediators or outside professionals—is a difficult call because outsiders, although more objective, may not grasp the on-site issues as well as someone who works in-house. On the other hand, an in-house colleague might not be skilled at mediation or might feel similarly threatened by the situation. The last desperate extreme, of course, is litigation against the supervisor and/or the company for inappropriate retaliation, discrimination, or termination, if it comes to that.

The whistleblower often walks a lonely road with many hazards, but his or her function is essential to uncovering hidden abuses within society. The risks of retaliation are sometimes, but not always, balanced by protections built into institutions and statutes so that this vital function can continue.

Ethical Commentary

By Penny Kyler, MA, OTR, FAOTA

Who Are the Players?

Ms. Wong, Mr. Donabedian, his daughter, his grandchild, Ms. Wong's supervisor, the interdisciplinary team, and other staff of the home health agency. Are there others?

What Other Information Is Needed?

What specifically has Ms. Wong told her supervisor? Where are Mr. Donabedian's daughter and grandchild? Have any other members of the interdisciplinary team raised similar concerns regarding Mr. Donabedian? Have any other members of the interdisciplinary team had similar concerns regarding the supervisor? What actions may be taken, and what are the possible consequences?

Concerns regarding reporting abuse almost always place individuals in ethical distress or in an ethical dilemma. To become involved or not to become involved? That is the question. Added to these concerns are, in some cases, cultural sensitivity issues. The classic case of the Hmong child whose parents used "cupping" to attempt to cure a seizure disorder as documented in Anne Fadiman's book, *The Spirit Catches You and You Fall Down,* graphically points out the collision of culture and medicine.

Is this a case in which cultural overtones need to be considered? Ms. Wong's action of attempting to talk to the daughter is a way of seeking the facts before acting. This is an important consideration because any accusation of abuse is serious, and steps in reporting such abuse should be taken prudently. Other needed information concerns individuals who act as whistleblowers; questions regarding how they will be perceived by their peers or supervisors should be asked. Ms. Wong's concerns regarding job security are very real. Some individuals have lost their jobs yet have persevered with the whistleblowing, and in the end have come away with their virtue and integrity intact, as well as back pay for dismissal without cause.

An occupational therapy practitioner may look to the Core Values and Attitudes of Occupational Therapy Practice (AOTA, 1993a), which states under the value of *truth* that practitioners should be faithful to facts and reality as they pertain to themselves and those they treat. The occupational therapy Code of Ethics (AOTA, 2000a) in Principles 1 and 2 embraces the ethical concepts of beneficence and nonmaleficence, admonishing all to do what is best for the client as well to avoid actions that may harm the client. Both of these concepts indicate that action should be taken when needed to make the therapeutic experience as positive as possible.

The Code indicates an active responsibility on the part of the occupational therapy practitioner to do something, thus as a member of the profession an obligation has been created. The Guidelines to the Occupational Therapy Code of Ethics (1998b) in Section 5.1 indicate that whereas practitioners should respect confidential information, if there is foreseeable or imminent hardship to a client, they have legal obligations to report such action. In all three documents, it is clear that the occupational therapy practitioner is expected to act in the best interests of the client.

Regarding the behavior of the supervisor and the fact that Ms. Wong believes that she smells alcohol on his breath, she needs to carefully consider whether she has an allegation or a fact. The smell of alcohol cannot be proven and therefore is an allegation and not a fact. The real or implied coercive nature of the supervisor's interactions with Ms. Wong is a point of concern. Ms. Wong may ask for a meeting with the supervisor to clarify what appears to be retaliation and, if possible, should have another person present as a witness, perhaps the human resource person at the agency. As an ethnic minority, Ms. Wong may take her concerns to the equal employment opportunity person at her work site. This individual may choose to handle her concerns or to refer her to another office outside the worksite. In either case, the impartial listener at the equal employment opportunity office should be able to provide some legal options for Ms. Wong to follow.

Conclusion

As noted in the commentary by Dr. Gutheil, whistleblowing occupies a special place in business and in health care. Whistleblowing inevitably poses some benefits as well as some problems to those involved. It places a burden on the individual who sets out to right a wrong; the person who tells people in authority things they often do not want to hear. The prudent person will look to guiding professional documents before acting. Clarify the facts and choose the best course of action for the client.

Study Questions

1. Why does a whistleblower emerge in a healthcare system?
2. Is there immunity for a whistleblower?
3. What are legal and ethical mandates for reporting?
4. What are some strategies the whistleblower can use to minimize the risks involved?
5. What protections exist within an institution to protect the whistleblower?

Glossary

Agreement of confidentiality—An understanding that sets forth the parameters of what information can be shared with a third party.

AIDS—Acquired immunodeficiency syndrome. The syndrome of opportunistic infections that occur as the final stage of infection by the human immunodeficiency virus (HIV) (Venes, Thomas, & Taber, 2001).

Antidiscrimination provisions of the ADA—Provisions the ADA has extended to all nonstate government employers with 15 or more employees, to state and local government services, and to all places of public accommodations regardless of whether they receive federal funds.

Apparent authority—When a person or entity allows another to appear to have the authority to act on his or her behalf, this person can be contractually bound.

Beneficience—Health professionals have a duty to act for the client's good.

Bioethics—A branch of ethics devoted to the study of problems surrounding medical practice, healthcare delivery, and medical and biological research.

Compensation—In record-keeping, the record provides accountability for work done (and omitted) for compensation by third-party payors, utilization review, and sometimes as a defense against charges of malpractice.

Competence—In informed consent, competence refers to the individual's capacity to weigh the information when processing a treatment decision.

Comprehensible—The third standard related to record-keeping is that the record should make long and complex treatment comprehensible.

Conduction—In physical agent modalities, the transfer of heat between two parts caused by a temperature difference between the parts.

Confidentiality—(In research) The expectation that information will not be divulged to others in ways that are inconsistent with the understanding of the original disclosure without permission (Office for the Protection from Research Risks Guidebook, 1993. Updated June 23, 2000).

Continuity—The record-keeping standard that refers to the fact that client care may take place over a long period with several caretakers. The record serves as an archive throughout the period of care.

Contractual obligation—A legally enforceable duty arising from a contract. The failure to abide by such an obligation can result in the damaged party seeking redress in the courts.

Convection—In physical agent modalities, refers to the transfer of heat by the circulation of heated parts of a liquid or gas.

Conversion—In physical agent modalities, refers to the transformation from one material or state to another.

Coordination—A record-keeping standard that means that all care providers move in the same direction with the client. The record permits sharing and coordination of information.

Countersigning—Countersigning treatment plans and notes in a client's record usually means the signer is taking on responsibility for the client.

Defamation—The offense of injuring a person's character, fame, or reputation by false and malicious statements. The term encompasses both libel and slander.

Disability—An individual with a disability is defined by the ADA as a person who has a physical or mental impairment that substantially limits major life activities; has a record of such impairment; or is regarded as having such impairment.

Disinterested party—(In whistleblowing) One who does not stand to be harmed or to benefit from exposing client or system abuse.

Doctrine of consent to treatment—A standard that physicians planning a treatment regimen or surgical procedure must obtain a patient's consent to do so; otherwise, the doctor is committing a battery, an unconsented touching.

Domain of concern—The unique area of expertise of a specific profession (Mosey, 1986, 1996).

Ethical dilemma—An ethical dilemma exists when no obvious satisfactory choice or answer is appropriate for a certain situation, or when there are only less-than-satisfactory alternatives.

Ethics—The careful and systematic study of the nature of morality.

Exposure-prone procedures—Invasive procedures including certain oral, cardiothoracic, colorectal, and obstetric/gynecologic procedures; general and orthopedic surgeries; and traumatic services. Interventions for dysphagia and scar management are considered exposure-prone procedures for occupational therapy practitioners.

Express contract—A contract in which parties have clearly stated their intentions.

Fieldwork site requirements—(In the ADA) The ADA lists the following requirements: (1) Fieldwork sites must integrate students with disabilities to the maximum extent appropriate. (2) Fieldwork sites must make reasonable modifications to their policies, practices, and procedures to accommodate persons with disabilities. (3) Fieldwork sites are also required to provide auxiliary aides and services to ensure effective communication with the student with a disability. (4) Fieldwork sites must remove architectural or other structural barriers in existing facilities to the extent that such steps are readily achievable.

Frame of reference—An organization of theoretical information that is grounded in a perspective that includes a conceptual rationale for various strategies or tools (Mosey, 1970, 1986, 1996).

Guardian—In law, one who acts as a vicarious decision maker on behalf of a person who has been found to be incompetent to make their own decisions.

HIV—Human immunodeficiency virus.

The HIV antibody test—It screens for antibodies associated with HIV. It does not screen for the AIDS virus. A positive test indicates only that an individual has been exposed to HIV but will not indicate if the virus is currently in the individual's system.

Human subject—(Now referred to as human participant) A person who consents to participate in a research investigation.

Impairment—Defined by the ADA as something that substantially limits major life activities.

Implied contract—A contract in which the conduct of parties is of paramount importance in determining whether a contract exists.

Informed consent—Consent containing three elements: information, voluntariness, and competence.

Informed consent emergencies—Special circumstances in which certain rules must be suspended to save life or prevent acute injury, deterioration, or similar harm.

Legal capacity—The age by which it is deemed that an individual (not suffering from severe mental or emotional impairment) can enter into binding contracts and other acts. This is frequently referred to as the "age of majority." In most jurisdictions in the United States, this age is 18 years.

Legal dilemma—A situation in which a full and equitable solution does not appear to be possible. There is no scientific right or wrong answer.

Libel—A form of defamation as expressed by print, writing, pictures, or signs. In its most general sense, libel includes any publication that is injurious to the reputation of another.

Major life activities—Defined by the ADA as functions such as caring for one's self, performing manual tasks, walking, seeing, hearing, speaking, breathing, learning, and working.

Mandated reporter—A healthcare worker or counselor who is required by law to report suspected abuse of protected groups such as children, elders, patients, or clients.

Mediation—(In whistleblowing) When an intermediary attempts to bring about a settlement between a whistleblower and someone higher in the hierarchy, usually so that no harm comes to the whistleblower, such as job loss.

Minimum Data Set (MDS)—OBRA defines the MDS as an interdisciplinary evaluative process that is completed with defined timelines.

Morality—A set of guidelines and standards that are striven for as ideals and that protect basic human values.

Nondiscrimination—Title III of the ADA enumerates three broad principles for nondiscrimination: (1) equal opportunity to participate, (2) equal opportunity to benefit, and (3) equal opportunity to receive benefits in the most integrated setting appropriate.

Nonmaleficence—The fundamental duty that instructs us not to do anything that would injure another.

Omnibus Budget Reconciliation Act—The Omnibus Budget Reconciliation Act (OBRA) is legislation addressing quality-of-care issues in nursing homes.

Physical agent modalities—Therapeutic agents that "use the properties of light, water, temperature, sound, and electricity to produce a response in soft tissue" (McGuire et al., 1991, p. 6).

Physical restraint—Defined by OBRA as any device attached or adjacent to one's body that restricts freedom of movement or normal access to one's body.

Privacy—(In research) Having control over the extent, timing, and circumstances of sharing oneself (physically, behaviorally, or intellectually) with others, in the context of a research study (Office for Protection from Research Risks Guidebook, 1993. Updated June 23, 2000).

Privacy Rule—(In research) As of April 2003, this law will require written permission by participants for their participation in a clinical trial or research and for use of their healthcare information in research.

Protections—(In whistleblowing) Laws and regulations that provide immunity for whistleblowers.

Public accommodation—Defined by the ADA as including but not limited to retail establishments, movie theaters, hospitals, hotels, doctor's offices, restaurants, and schools.

Quasi-contracts—Contracts in which the parties fail to conform to contractual prerequisites, but justice requires an obligation of payment. These are not considered legal contracts but rather situations in which the absence of payment or compensation would be manifestly unjust. Only a court of law can make such a determination based on the merits of each case.

Readily achievable—Defined by the ADA as changes that are easily accomplishable and able to be carried out without much difficulty or expense.

Reasonable payment—In law, compensation deemed to be sufficient and appropriate under the given circumstances by the custom and practice in a given geographic or metropolitan area.

Relative benefit—In healthcare ethics, a consideration to forego some greater benefit for some clients who start out much better off in order to produce a lesser benefit for clients who start out worse off.

Resident Assessment Instrument (RAI)—OBRA dictates that an assessment of a nursing home resident (RAI) must include the resident's: medical history, current medical status, functional status, sensory and physical impairments, nutritional status and requirements, special treatments and procedures, psychosocial status, discharge potential, dental condition, activities potential, rehabilitation potential, cognitive status, and drug therapy.

Retaliation—(In whistleblowing) Retribution or revenge a whistleblower may experience in response to reporting suspected abuse.

Shotgun approach—In healthcare ethics, a plan that gives everybody a chance at some benefit versus one that produces a big benefit for a smaller number of people.

Slander—The verbal form of defamation. The speaking of false and malicious words concerning another, whereby injury results to the subject's reputation.

Specific competence—A person may be deemed incompetent in one or more specific areas while still being able to participate in other decisions.

Thermal modalities—In physical agent modalities, methods of heat transfer that include conduction, convection, and conversion.

Third-party payor—A source of funding beyond the immediate recipient of service: from the individual, to the insurer, to the payor of services.

Tools—(In healthcare professions) The items, means, methods, and instruments that are used in practice in a theoretically proscribed manner to bring about change.

Universal Precautions—The appropriate use of hand washing, protective barriers, and care in the use and disposal of needles and other sharp instruments.

Utilitarianism—The doctrine that advocates doing the most good for the highest number of people.

Utility—Behave in ways that will result in the greatest benefit and the least harm.

Vicarious liability—The way an individual may be liable for the actions of another, usually a supervisee.

Whistleblower—One who brings to the attention of authorities a person he or she believes may be causing harm to a child, elder, patient, or client, or who one may be abusing the system.

References

Accreditation Council for Occupational Therapy Education. (1999a). Standards for an accredited educational program for the occupational therapist. *American Journal of Occupational Therapy, 53*, 575–582.

Accreditation Council for Occupational Therapy Education. (1999b). Standards for an accredited education program for the occupational therapy assistant. *American Journal of Occupational Therapy, 53*, 583–589.

American Dental Association. (1991). *ADA policy on HIV-infected dentists.* Chicago: Author.

American Occupational Therapy Association. (1979). Policy I.12: Occupation as the Common Core of Occupational Therapy. In *Policy manual of the American Occupational Therapy Association.* Rockville, MD: Author.

American Occupational Therapy Association. (1989a). *Human immunodeficiency virus* (position paper). Rockville, MD: Author.

American Occupational Therapy Association. (1989b November). *Report from the legal affairs division.* Rockville, MD: Author.

American Occupational Therapy Association. (1991). AOTA statement on physical agent modalities. *American Journal of Occupational Therapy, 45,* 1075.

American Occupational Therapy Association. (1993a). Core values and attitudes of occupational therapy practice. *American Journal of Occupational Therapy, 47,* 1085–1086.

American Occupational Therapy Association. (1993b). Occupational therapy roles. *American Journal of Occupational Therapy, 47,* 1087–1099.

American Occupational Therapy Association. (1995). Occupational therapy: A profession in support of full inclusion. *American Journal of Occupational Therapy, 49,* 1009.

American Occupational Therapy Association. (1997). Position Paper: Physical agent modalities. *American Journal of Occupational Therapy, 51,* 870–871.

American Occupational Therapy Association. (1998a). Standards of Practice for Occupational Therapy. *American Journal of Occupational Therapy, 52,* 866–869.

American Occupational Therapy Association. (1998b). Guidelines to the occupational therapy code of ethics. *American Journal of Occupational Therapy, 52,* 881–884.

American Occupational Therapy Association (1999a). Occupational therapy's commitment to nondiscrimination and inclusion. *American Journal of Occupational Therapy, 53,* 598.

American Occupational Therapy Association. (1999b). Standards for continuing competence. *American Journal of Occupational Therapy, 53,* 599–600.

American Occupational Therapy Association. (2000a). Occupational therapy code of ethics. *American Journal of Occupational Therapy, 54,* 614–616.

American Occupational Therapy Association. (2000b). Enforcement procedures for Occupational Therapy Code of Ethics. *American Journal of Occupational Therapy, 54,* 617–621.

American Occupational Therapy Association. (2002). Occupational therapy practice framework: Domain and process. *American Journal of Occupational Therapy, 56,* 607–637.

American Psychological Association Practice Organization. (Winter 2002). Special HIPAA compliance issue: Practitioner focus, 14(1).

Americans with Disabilities Act, Pub. L. No. 101–336 (1990) 42 U.S.C. 12101 et seq.

Bayer, R., Levine, C., & Wolf, S. (1986). HIV antibody screening: An ethical framework for evaluating proposed programs. *Journal of the American Medical Association, 256,* 634–638.

Beauchamp, T. L., & Childress, J. F. (1994). *Principles of biomedical ethics* (4th ed.). New York: Oxford University Press.

Beauchamp, T. L., & Walters, L. (Eds.). (1989). *Contemporary issues in bioethics* (3rd ed). Belmont, CA: Wadsworth.

Black, H. C. (1968). *Black's law dictionary* (4th ed.). St. Paul, MN: West Publishing.

Blatchford, O., O'Brien, S. J., Blatchford, M., & Taylor, A. (2000). Infectious health care workers: Should patients be told? *Journal of Medical Ethics, 26,* 27–33.

Board of Trustees of the University of Alabama v. *Garrett,* 531 U.S. 356, 121 S.Ct. 955 (2001).

Bracciano, A. G., & Earley, D. (2002). Physical agent modalities. In C. A. Trombly and M. V. Radmonski, *Occupational therapy for physical dysfunction* (5th ed.) (pp. 421–441). Baltimore: Lippincott, Williams & Williams.

Breines, E. B. (2001). Therapeutic occupations and modalities. In L. W. Pedretti and M. B. Early, *Occupational therapy: Practice skills for physical dysfunction* (2nd ed.) (pp. 519–525). Philadelphia: Mosby.

Centers for Disease Control. (1988). *Perspectives in disease prevention and health promotion update: Universal precautions for prevention of transmission of human immunodeficiency virus, hepatitis B virus, and other blood-borne pathogens in health care settings.* Morbidity and mortality weekly report 37 (24); 377–388. Atlanta: U.S. Department of Health and Human Services. Available from Centers for Disease Control Website, www.cdc.gov/mmwr/preview/mmwrhtml/00000039.htm.

Centers for Disease Control. (1991). *Recommendations for preventing transmission of human immunodeficiency virus and hepatitis B virus to patients during exposure prone invasive procedures.* Morbidity and mortality weekly report 40 (No. RR-8); 1–9. Atlanta: U.S. Department of Health and Human

Services. Available from Centers for Disease Control Website, www.cdc.gov/mmwr/preview/mmwrhtml/00014845.htm.

Centers for Disease Control and Prevention (1999). *Guidelines for national immunodeficiency virus case surveillance, including monitoring for human immunodeficiency virus infection and acquired immunodeficiency syndrome.* Morbidity and mortality weekly report 48 (No. RR-13); 1–28. Atlanta: U.S. Department of Health and Human Services. Available from the Centers for Disease Control Website, www.cdc.gov/mmwr/preview/mmwrhtml/rr4813a1.htm.

Centers for Disease Control and Prevention (2001a). *HIV Prevention Strategic Plan Through 2005.* Atlanta: U.S. Department of Health and Human Services. Available from the Centers for Disease Control Website, www.cdc.gov/hiv/pubs/prev-strat-plan.pdf.

Centers for Disease Control and Prevention (2001b). *Updated U.S. Public Health Service guidelines for the management of occupational exposures to HBV, HCV, & HIV and recommendations for postexposure prophylaxis.* Morbidity and mortality weekly report 50 (No. RR-11); 1–42. Atlanta: U.S. Department of Health and Human Services. Available from the Centers for Disease Control Website, www.cdc.gov/mmwr/PDF/rr/rr5011.pdf.

Centers for Disease Control and Prevention (2002a). *Preventing occupational HIV transmission to healthcare personnel.* Available from Centers for Disease Control Website, www.cdc.gov/hiv/pubs/facts/hcwprev.htm.

Centers for Disease Control and Prevention (2002b). *Surveillance of healthcare workers with HIV/AIDS.* Available from Centers for Disease Control Website, www.cdc.gov/hiv/pubs/facts/hcwsurv.htm.

Chevron U.S.A. Inc. v. Echazabal, _____ U.S. _____, 122 S.Ct. 2045 (2002).

Civil Rights Restoration Act, Pub. L. No. 100–259 (1988).

Code of Federal Regulations, Title 45 Public Welfare, Department of Health and Human Services, National Institutes of Health, Office for Protection from Research Risks. Part 46. Protection of Human Subjects. Revised June 18, 1991. Effective August 19, 1991.

Code of Federal Regulations, Title 21, Food and Drug Administration. Volume 1, Parts 50 and 56. Revised April 1, 2000.

Comer, R. W., Myers, D. R., Steadman, C. D., Carter, M. J., Rissing, J. D., & Tedesco, F. J. (1991). Management considerations for an HIV positive dental student. *Journal of Dental Education, 55(3),* 187–191.

Curtin, L., & Flaherty, J. M. (1999). *Nursing ethics: Theories and pragmatics.* Stamford, CT: Appleton & Lange.

Dunbar, J. M., Neufeld, R. R., White, H. C., & Libow, L. S. (1996). Retrain, don't restrain: The educational intervention of the national nursing home restraint removal project. *Gerontologist, 36,* 539–542.

Education of the Handicapped Act, Pub. L. No. 94–142 (1975).

Elon, R., & Pawlson, L. G. (1992). The impact of OBRA on medical practice within nursing facilities. *Journal of the American Geriatric Society, 40,* 958–963.

Emanuel, E. J., & Emanuel, L. L. (1992). Four models of physician patient relationships. *Journal of the American Medical Association, 267,* 2221–2226.

Equal Employment Opportunity Commission. *1992 Title I technical assistance manual.* Washington, DC: U.S. Government Printing Office.

Evans, L., & Strumpf, N. (1989). Tying down the elderly: A review of the literature on physical restraint. *Journal of the American Geriatric Society, 37,* 65–74.

Fadiman, A. (1997). *The spirit catches you and you fall down: A Hmong child, her American doctors and the collision of two cultures.* New York: Farrar, Strauss & Giroux.

Fidler, G. S. (1992). Letter to the editor: Against the use of physical agent modalities. *American Journal of Occupational Therapy, 46,* 567–568.

Friedland, G. H., & Klein, R. S. (1987). Transmission of the human immunodeficiency virus. *New England Journal of Medicine, 317,* 1125–1135.

Gaston v. Belhingrath Garden & Home, Inc., 167 F.3d 1361, 11th Cir. (1999).

Gifis, S. (1984). *Law dictionary.* New York: Barron's Educational Services.

Gilligan, C. (1982). *In a different voice: Psychological theory and women's development.* Cambridge, MA: Harvard University Press.

Gostin, L. (1989, January/February). HIV-infected physicians and the practice of seriously invasive procedures, *Hastings Center Report,* pp. 32–59.

Hansen, R. A., Kamp, L., & Reitz, S. (1988). Two practitioners' analysis of occupational therapy. *American Journal of Occupational Therapy, 42,* 312–319.

Hansen, R., & Kyler-Hutchison, P. (1989). *Light at the end of the tunnel.* Workshop at the Annual Conference of the American Occupational Therapy Association, Baltimore, MD.

Hansen, R., & Kyler-Hutchison, P. (1992). Ethical considerations for the consultant. In A. Aroskar, E. Jaffe, & C. Epstein (Eds.), *Occupational therapy consultation: Theory, principles and practice* (Chapter 39). St. Louis: C. V. Mosby.

Health Care Financing Administration. (1989). State operations manual. Department of Health and Human Services, Transmittal No. 232.

Health Care Financing Administration. (1992). State operations manual. Department of Health and Human Services, Transmittal No. 250, pp. 76–78.

Hemelt, M. D., & Mackert, M. E. (1978). *Dynamics of law in nursing and health care.* Englewood Cliffs, NJ: Prentice Hall.

Hilts, P. (1991, October 4). Congress urges AIDS tests for doctors. *New York Times,* p. A8.

Hinojosa, J., Bowen, R., Case-Smith, J., Epstein, C. F., Moyers, P., & Schwope, C. (2000a). Self-initiated continuing competence. *OT Practice, 5*(24), CE1–CE8.

Hinojosa, J., Bowen, R., Case-Smith, J., Epstein, C. F., Moyers, P., & Schwope, C. (2000b). Self-study: Standards for continuing competence for occupational therapy practitioners. *OT Practice, 5*(7), CE1–CE8.

Hopp, J.W., & Rogers, E.A. (1989). *AIDS and the allied health professions.* Philadelphia: F.A. Davis.

Jaffee, S., & Hyde, J. S. (2000). Gender differences in moral orientation: A meta-analysis. *Psychological Bulletin, 126,* 703–726.

Jaffee v. Redmond, 518 U.S. 1 (1996).

Janelli, L. M., Kanski, G. W., & Neary, M. A. (1994). Physical restraints: Has OBRA made a difference? *Journal of Gerontological Nursing, 20*(6), 17–21.

Kail, R. V. (1998). *Children and their development.* Upper Saddle River, NJ: Prentice Hall.

Koelbl, J. J. (1992, March). *The HIV positive dental student: Are we prepared to act with care and compassion?* Paper presented at the American Association of Dental Schools, Boston, MA.

Kohlberg, L. (1963). The development of children's orientation toward a moral order: 1 – Sequence in the development of moral thought. *Vita Humana, 6,* pp. 11–33.

Kohlberg, L. (1964). Development of moral character and moral ideology. In M. L. Hoffman & L. W. Hoffman (Eds.), *Review of Child Development Research*, Vol. 1. New York: Russell Sage Foundation.

Kohlberg, L. (1969). Stage and sequence: The cognitive-developmental approach to socialization. In D. A. Goslin (Ed.), *Handbook of socialization: Theory and research*, pp. 347–480. Chicago: Rand McNally.

Kramer, P., & Hinojosa, J. (Eds.). (1993). *Frames of reference for pediatric occupational therapy.* Baltimore, MD: Williams & Wilkins.

Luebben, A. J., Hinojosa, J., & Kramer, P. (1999). Legitimate tools of pediatric occupational therapy. In P. Kramer & J. Hinojosa (Eds.), *Frames of reference for pediatric occupational therapy* (pp. 27–40). Baltimore: Lippincott, Williams & Wilkins.

Martelli, L. J., Peltz, C. R. C., & Messina, W. (1987). *When someone you know has AIDS: A practical guide.* New York: Crown Publishers.

McGuire, M. J. et al. (1991). *Physical agent modality task group report.* Rockville, MD: AOTA.

Michlovitz, S. (1991). *Thermal agents in rehabilitation.* Philadelphia: F. A. Davis.

Miike, L., Ostrowsky, J., Bahney, C., & Hewitt, PM. (1991). *HIV in the heath care workplace.* Washington, DC: Office of Technology Assessment at the Congress of the United States.

Miles, S. H., & Myers, R. (1994). Untying the elderly: 1989 to 1993 update. *Clinics in Geriatric Medicine, 10*, 513–525.

Milliken, N., & Greenblatt, R. (1988). Ethical issues of the AIDS epidemic. In J. F. Monagle & D. Thomasma (Eds.), *Medical ethics: A guide for health professionals* (pp. 443–459). Rockville, MD: Aspen Publishers.

Morisky v. *Broward County*, 80 F.3d 445 (1996).

Mosey, A. C. (1970). *Three frames of reference for mental health.* Thorofare, NJ: Slack.

Mosey, A. C. (1986). *Psychosocial components of occupational therapy.* New York: Raven Press.

Mosey. A. C. (1996). *Applied scientific inquiry in the health professions: An epistemological orientation* (2nd ed.). Bethesda, MD: AOTA.

Munson, R. (1988). *Intervention and reflection: Basic issues in medical ethics* (3rd ed.). Belmont, CA: Wadsworth Publishing Company.

Neistadt, M. E., & Crepeau, E. B. (Eds.). (1998). *Willard and Spackman's occupational therapy.* Philadelphia: J.B. Lippincott.

O'Rourke, K. D., & de Blois, J. (1991). The right to know: Ethical issues related to mandatory testing of healthcare workers for HIV. *Health Progress*, pp. 39–43.

Percesepe, G. (1995). *Introduction to ethics: Personal and social responsibility in a diverse world.* Englewood, NJ: Prentice Hall.

Pizzi, M. (1990). Nationally speaking: The transformation of HIV infection and AIDS in occupational therapy: Beginning the conversation. *American Journal of Occupational Therapy, 44*, 199–203.

Pizzi, M., & Burkhardt, A. (1998). Occupational therapy for adults with immunological diseases. In M. E. Neistadt & E. B. Crepeau (Eds.), *Willard and Spackman's occupational therapy.* (9th ed.) (p. 712). Philadelphia: J.B. Lippincott.

Purtilo, P. (1989). *Ethics in professional practice.* American Occupational Therapy Practice Symposium. Rockville, MD: AOTA.

Rehabilitation Act, Pub. L. No. 93–516 (1973), Section 504. Amended 29 U.S.C. 794.

Rennert, S. (1991). *AIDS/HIV and confidentiality. Model policy and procedures.* Washington, DC: American Bar Association.

Roberts v. *Gonzaga University,* U.S. S.Ct. No.01–679 (2001).

Ross, D. (1988). Basic theories in medical ethics. In J. F. Monagle & D. Thomasma (Eds.), *Medical ethics: A guide for health professionals* (pp. 468–483). Rockville, MD: Aspen Publishers.

Rotary International. (1990). *Applying the four-way test.* Chicago: Author.

Rutan, J. S., & Stone, W. N. (1984). *Psychodynamic group psychotherapy.* Lexington, MA: D. C. Heath & Company.

Shin et al. v. *M.I.T. et al.* Middx. Sup. Ct., Civil Action No. 02–0403 (2002).

Simpson, L. P. (1965). *Law of contracts* (2nd ed.). St. Paul, MN: West Publishing.

Southeastern Community College v. *Davis,* 442 U.S. 2361 (1979).

Sultz, H. A., & Young, K. M. (2001). *Healthcare USA: Understanding its organization and delivery.* Gaithersburg, MD: Aspen Publications.

Tinetti, M. E., Liu, W. L., Maratolli, A. R., & Ginter, S. F. (1991). Mechanical restraint use among residents of skilled nursing facilities: Prevalence, patterns and predictors. *Journal of the American Medical Association, 265,* 468–471.

Toyota Motor Mfg., Kentucky, Inc. v. *Williams,* 534 U.S. 184, 122 S.Ct. 681 (2002).

Trombly, C. A. (Ed.). (1982). Include exercise in purposeful activity. (Letter to the editor). *American Journal of Occupational Therapy, 36,* 467–468.

U.S. Department of Education, Office for Civil Rights. (1989). *The rights of individuals with handicaps under federal law.* Washington, DC: U.S. Government Printing Office.

U.S. Department of Justice. (1992). *Title III Technical Assistance Manual.* Washington DC: U.S. Government Printing Office.

Venes, D., Thomas, C., & Taber, C.W. (Eds.) (2001). *Taber's cyclopedic medical dictionary* (19th ed.). Philadelphia: F.A. Davis.

Wallerstein, R. S. (1976). Introduction to symposium on "Ethics, moral values and psychological interventions." *International Review of Psycho-Analysis, 3,* 369–372.

Weinstein, B. D., & Keyes, O. (1991). Management considerations for an HIV positive dental student: Ethical and legal commentary. *Journal of Dental Education, 55,* 238–240.

Weiss, S. H. (1992). HIV infection and the health care worker. *Medical Clinics of North America, 7(1),* 269–280.

Wendell, S. (1992). Towards a feminist theory of disability. In H. B. Holmes & L. M. Purdy (Eds.), *Feminist perspectives in edical ethics.* Bloomington, IN: Indiana University Press.

Additional Reading

Ackerman, T. F., & Strong, C. (1989). *A casebook of medical ethics.* New York: Oxford University Press.

Bayer, R., Caplan, A., & Daniels, N. (Eds.). (1983). *In search of equity: Health needs and the health care system.* New York: Plenum Press.

Behnke, S. H., & Hilliard, J. T. (1998). *The essentials of Massachusetts mental health law.* New York: Norton.

Benjamin, M., & Curtin, S. (1986). *Ethics in nursing* (2nd ed.). New York: Oxford University Press.

Cotton, P. (1989). Confidentiality: A sacred trust under siege. *Medical World News, 30(6),* 54–57.

Emanuel, E. (1991). *The ends of human life: Medical ethics in a liberal polity.* Cambridge: Cambridge University Press.

Gelfman, M. H., & Schwab, N. C. (1991). School health services and educational records: Conflicts in the law. *West's Education Law Report, 64(2),* 319–328.

Gutheil, T. G. (1997). The medical record in the acute care setting and issues of confidentiality. In L. I. Sederer and A. J. Rothschild (Eds.), *Acute care psychiatry: Diagnosis and treatment.* Baltimore: Williams & Wilkins.

Gutheil, T. G., & Applebaum, P. S. (2000). *Clinical handbook of psychiatry and the law* (3rd ed.). Baltimore: Lippincott, Williams & Wilkins.

Hansen, R. A. (1988). Special issue on ethics. *American Journal of Occupational Therapy, 42,* 279–319.

Joseph, D., & Onek, J. (1991). Confidentiality in psychiatry. In P. Chodoff & S. Block (Eds.), *Psychiatric ethics* (pp. 313–340). Oxford: Oxford University Press.

Index

Page numbers followed by "t" indicate tables.

A

"Above all, do no harm," 6

Abuse
child, sexual, and spousal, 127
elder, 192

Accommodations
for equal access, 14
public, 36, 37, 40, 46, 49
reasonable, 47, 48, 49, 50–51, 74–75
See also Architectural and structural
barriers

Accreditation Council for Occupational
Therapy (ACOTE), Standards for an
Accredited Educational Program,
104

Accreditation requirements, 10

ACOTE. *See* Accreditation Council for
Occupational Therapy

Acquired immunodeficiency syndrome
(AIDS), 127, 148, 197
confidentiality rights, 158
education programs, 160
incidence and prevalence of, 59–60
screening for, 8
See also Human immunodeficiency
virus (HIV)

Acquired immunodeficiency syndrome
(AIDS)-related complex (ARC), 152

Active versus passive processes, 102, 103

ADA. *See* Americans with Disabilities
Act

Adaptive equipment, 43, 185, 186

Adversarial situations, 57

Age of majority, 179

Age and use of restraints, 117

Agency law, 181, 184

Agreement of confidentiality, 125, 131,
132, 197

Agreement memorandum, 61–62

AIDS. *See* Acquired immunodeficiency
syndrome

Ajouelo v. Auto-Soler Co., 25

Alternatives to restraints, 116, 119, 120t,
122

Alzheimer's disease, 153, 158–159, 161

Ambiguity and contracts, 178, 184–185

Amdur, Robert and Bankert, Elizabeth,
"Institutional Review Board
Management and Function," 167

American Bar Association, 73

American Dental Association, 69

American Hospital Association, 69

American Occupational Therapy
Association (AOTA)
Commission on Education, 54
Core Values and Attitudes of
Occupational Therapy Practice, 29,
44, 56, 194
Occupational Therapy Practice
Framework: Domain and Process, 102
Occupational Therapy Roles, 95–96
Representative Assembly on physical
agent modalities (1991), 99
Standards for Continuing Competence,
104, 105

American Occupational Therapy
Association (AOTA) Code of Ethics,
28–29, 32
autonomy, 9
beneficence, 5–6

American Occupational Therapy
(Continued)
Common Rule, 134, 167
confidentiality, 63
Enforcement Procedures for, 9
ethical analysis, 45
fieldwork supervisors, 51–52, 55, 57
fraud, 93–94
Guidelines to, 9, 29, 44, 54, 56, 95, 96,
110, 167, 173, 185–186, 194
and HIV, 62
nonmaleficence, 6
preamble to, 131
Principle 1), 93, 122, 161, 194
Principle 2), 72, 110, 187, 194
Principle 3), 56, 93, 94, 105, 110, 173
Principle 4), 96, 105, 109–110
Principle 5), 46, 93, 94, 95
Principle 7), 63, 131
social responsibility, 186
teaching about, 30
*American Occupational Therapy
Association (AOTA) Position
Statement on Occupational
Therapy's Commitment to
Nondiscrimination and Inclusion,*
80
American Occupational Therapy
Association (AOTA) Standards of
Practice, 29, 37, 44, 105
confidentiality, 46
ethical analysis, 45
fieldwork supervisors, 51–52
obligations of therapists, 47
social responsibility, 186
Americans with Disabilities Act (ADA),
13, 34–57
antidiscrimination provisions, 37
architectural and structural barriers, 43
auxiliary aides and services, 43, 49
definition of disability, 38, 40–41
eligibility criteria, 42
ethical analysis, 45–53
emotional problems on fieldwork
placement case study, 34–35,
46–49, 53–57
physical disability on fieldwork
placement case study, 35, 49–52,
53–57
ethics and the law, 44–45
fieldwork site requirements, 42
nondiscrimination principles, 41–42
outside contracts, 44
policy modifications, 42–43
public accommodations, 36, 37, 40,
46, 49
purpose of, 36–37

reasonable accommodation, 47, 48, 49,
50–51, 74–75
safety requirements, 44
Title III, 40, 45, 48, 49, 52
Titles I and II, 39–40, 50
See also Section 504 of the
Rehabilitation Act of 1973
Anonymous testing centers for HIV, 65
Antidiscrimination provisions of the
Americans with Disabilities Act
(ADA), 37, 197
Antipsychotic medication, 156
Antiretroviral therapy, 60
AOTA. *See* American Occupational
Therapy Association (AOTA)
Apparent authority, 181, 182, 197
ARC. *See* Acquired immunodeficiency
syndrome (AIDS)-related complex
Architectural and structural barriers, 43
See also Accommodations
Aroskar, A., 45
Assessment
interdisciplinary, 119
nursing home Resident Assessment
Instrument (RAI)/Minimum Data Set
(MDS), 114–115
nursing home Resident Assessment
Protocols (RAPs), 115, 116t
Assistive devices, 103
Autonomy, principle of, 8–9, 73, 84, 120,
121, 134, 154
Auxiliary aides and services, 43, 49

B
Bailey, Diana, 137–151
Barriers in contact with blood or body
fluids, 68
Bartering, 186, 188
Behavioral symptoms and use of
restraints, 117, 119
Beneficence, principle of, 4–6, 83, 134,
197
Best-off/worst-off clients. *See* Sick/sicker
clients
Bias, unconscious, 14
Billable treatments, 92
"Bills of rights," 157
Bioethics, 3–4, 197
Bipolar disorder and ARC case study,
152–163, 157–158, 159–160
Blood donations, 64
Bloodborne pathogens, 66, 67
*Board of Trustees of the University of
Alabama v. Garrett,* 37
Boundary issues, 125, 128, 129, 130, 131
Braille materials, 43
Breach of contract, 17, 26

Buckley Amendment. *See* Family Educational Rights and Privacy Act

C

Carbamazepine, 155
Care orientation, 2
Career counseling, 74
Caregiver support group case study. *See* Support group case study
Carelessness, 6
Case analysis format for resolution of ethical dilemmas, 28–33
Case finders, 158
Case law, 44, 156
Centers for Disease Control and Prevention (CDC)
epidemiologic survey programs, 67–68
HIV case study, 59, 62, 68, 70, 71
national hotline for AIDS information, 65
Universal Precautions for Prevention and Transmission of HIV, HBV, and Other Bloodborne Pathogens in Health Care Settings, 66
Centers for Medicare and Medicaid Services (CMS), 114, 121
Certification procedures, 6, 137
Certification requirements, 61, 76
Chaiklin, Harris, 130
Cheating case study, 13, 15–32
Chemistry courses, 106
Chevron U.S.A. Inc. v. Echazabal, 50
Child abuse, 127
Chronic mental disorders, 159
CITI. *See* Collaborative IRB Training Initiative
Civil liability, 191
Civil liberties, 22
Civil rights, 36, 74
Civil Rights Restoration Act (1988), 38
Civil statutes, 4
Clarity in contracts, 184–185
Client-centered care, 160
Client function versus discomfort (case), 11–12
Client record, 83, 85–96
case studies, 83, 85–96
documentation pitfalls, 90–91
documentation principles, 88–89
client's capacity to contribute, 88, 89
exercise of clinical judgment at decision points, 88, 89
risk-benefit analysis, 88–89
liability context, 87
risk management approach, 83, 87
roles of the record, 87
signatures and record-keeping, 91–92

See also Documentation; Records
Clients
"Above all, do no harm," 6
"bills of rights," 157
capacity to contribute, 88, 89
dangerousness of, 134, 156
decision making by, 56–57
direct threat to, 49–51
doctrine of consent to treatment, 154
fidelity to, 94, 110
HIV case study, 71–75
informed consent in research case study, 164–175
obligation to potential, 143–144
protection of, 13
quality of care, 64
relatives of, 138
right to refuse treatment, 57, 110, 134, 152, 155–157
risk to, 63
safe care of, 55–56, 57
Clinical decision making, 118–119
Clinical judgment at decision points, 88, 89
Clinical practice, ethical and legal dilemmas in, 3
Clinical supervisors, 46
Clinicians, 83–84
client record case studies, 83, 85–96
making choices, 144
physical agent modalities case study, 83–84, 97–111
restraints in the nursing home case study, 84, 112–123
support group case study, 84
See also Supervisors
Closed-captioned videotapes, 43
CMS. *See* Centers for Medicare and Medicaid Services
Code of Ethics. *See* American Occupational Therapy Association (AOTA) Code of Ethics
Code of Federal Regulations, 166, 168
Code of the Food and Drug Administration, 166
Cognitive impairment and use of restraints, 117, 119
Cohn, Ellen S., 77
Cold packs as physical therapeutic agent, 99
Collaborative IRB Training Initiative (CITI), 170
Commitment/treatment schism, 155–156
Common Rule, 134, 166, 167, 169, 170, 171
Communication, 43

Community practice standards, 95
Comparative justice, principle of, 7
Compensation by third-party payors, 88, 197
Competence, 92, 152
 continuing, 104, 108
 and informed consent, 152, 154–155, 197
 physical agent modalities case study, 105–107
 specific, 162
 testing for, 161–163
Competing needs of society, 7, 133
Comprehensible standard in client record, 88, 197
Computers, 22
Conduction, 99–100, 101t, 197
Confidentiality, 9, 13, 197
 agreement of, 125, 131, 132
 defined legally, 127
 of educational records, 46
 and HIV, 60, 62–63, 64, 65, 71, 73, 78, 159
 informed consent in research case study, 168, 169, 171, 172
 of records, 14, 22–23
 in support and therapy groups, 84
 in whistleblowing, 192
 See also Support group case study
Consumer advocacy groups, 113
Consumer-oriented society, 109, 121
Continuing competence, 104, 108
Continuity standard in client record, 87, 198
Contract, breach of, 17, 26
Contract law, 178–180, 184
Contracts, 176–188
 acceptance or rejection of the offer, 182
 age of majority, 179, 180
 agency law, 181, 184
 and ambiguity, 178, 184–185
 apparent authority, 181, 182
 case study, 176–177
 clarity of, 184–185
 contract law, 178–180, 184
 contractual obligation, 178
 counteroffer, 180, 182
 customary practice, 183
 definition, 178
 elements of a contract, 180–183
 express contracts, 179–180, 183, 184
 implied contracts (implied-in-fact), 179, 180, 184
 legal capacity, 179, 180
 legal consideration, 179
 legality of subject matter, 179
 mutual assent, 179, 180

quasi-contracts (implied-in-law), 180, 184
 reasonable payment, 183, 184
 true contracts, 179
 verbal agreements, 179
 written contracts, 178, 184
Contractual obligation, 178, 198
Contrast baths as physical therapeutic agent, 99
Contribution, principle of, 8
Convection, 99–100, 101t, 198
Conversion, 99–100, 101t, 198
Coordination standard in client record, 87, 198
Core Values and Attitudes of Occupational Therapy Practice. *See* American Occupational Therapy Association (AOTA) Core Values and Attitudes of Occupational Therapy Practice
Costs of health care, 4
Counseling
 career, 74
 and HIV, 64–66
Counteroffer in contracts, 180, 182
Countersigning, 91, 198
Couples therapy, 127
Credentialing trainees, 92
Creed (civil rights protection), 36
Criminal statutes, 4
Cryotherapy as physical therapeutic agent, 99
Cultural heritage, 160–161, 162
Custodial care, 147
Customary practice, 134, 183
 See also Reasonable and accepted practice

D
Daily life activities, 102, 119, 161
Dana Farber Cancer Research Center (Boston), 137
Dangerous clients, 134
Daniels, Norman, 133, 135–151
Decision making, 133
 by clients, 56–57
 proxy, 119
Decision-making process, 2, 29
Decision points, clinical judgment at, 88, 89
Defamation, 17, 19, 21, 27, 198
 libel, 26
 slander, 26
Deliberative model of care, 160
Dental workers, 60, 68, 69, 74
Deontologic point of view, 94–95
Dependent children status, 25

Diagnostic related groups (DRGs), 52
Dilemmas
  definition of, 29
  See also Ethical dilemmas; Legal
    dilemmas
Directory information, 22
Disability
  definition, 38, 40–41, 198
  See also Americans with Disabilities
    Act (ADA); Students, with disabilities
Discrimination, 13, 36, 48, 49
  by employers in whistleblowing,
    191–192, 193
  and HIV, 64
Disinterested parties in whistleblowing,
  191, 198
Distributive justice, principle of, 7–8, 14
Doctrine of consent to treatment, 154,
  198
Documentation, 83
  documentation for reimbursement case
    study, 85–86, 90, 92–95
  pitfalls in, 89–91
  principles of, 88–89
  in whistleblowing, 192–193
  See also Client record; Records
Domain of concern of a profession,
  101–103, 198
Domain of practice, 83
DRGs. *See* Diagnostic related groups
Drug testing, 3
Dual relationships, 128
"Due care" standards, 6

E
Education of the Handicapped Act (1975),
  36
Educational background, physical agent
  modalities, 103–105, 106
Educational "goods," 14
Educational records, 25, 46
Educational training, 104
EEOC. *See* Equal Employment
  Opportunity Commission
Effort, principle of, 8
Elderly care facilities. *See* Nursing homes
Elderly people, 160–161
  abuse of, 192
  See also Family imposes treatment on
    relative; Restraints in the nursing
    home case study
Electrical stimulation as physical
  therapeutic agent, 99
Eligibility criteria, 42
Emanuel, Ezekiel, 133, 135–151
Emergency exception to informed
  consent, 155

Emotional problems in fieldwork
  placement case study, 34–35,
  46–49, 53–57
Emotional stability, 63–64
Employment, 36
Engagement in meaningful occupations
  and activities, 186
English common law, 179
Entrenched policy, 190
Entry-level practice, 104, 107, 173
Environmental adaptations, 119, 120
Environmental assessment, 121, 148
Equal access, accommodations for, 14
Equal Employment Opportunity
  Commission (EEOC), 50, 195
Equal opportunity to benefit, 41–42
Equal opportunity to participate, 40,
  41–42
Equal opportunity to receive benefits in
  the most integrated setting
  appropriate, 41–42
Equal rights, 36
Equality, principle of, 8
Equipment operation and care, 106
Ervin, Sam, 21, 22
Essential job functions, 51
Ethical analysis, 45–53
  emotional problems on fieldwork
    placement case study, 34–35, 46–49,
    53–57
  physical disability on fieldwork
    placement case study, 35, 49–52,
    53–57
Ethical dilemmas, 2–4, 198
  case analysis format for resolution of,
    28–33
  Human immunodeficiency virus
    (HIV), 60
  support group case study, 125, 128–129
Ethical principles, 4–9, 29
  autonomy, 8–9
  beneficence, 4–6
  comparative justice, 7
  contribution, 8
  distributive justice, 7–8
  effort, 8
  equality, 8
  need, 8
  noncomparative justice, 7
  nonmaleficence, 6
  utility, 6–7
Ethical subjectivism, 132
Ethics, 3, 126, 198
  ethical subjectivism, 132
  and the law, 44–45
  social contract ethics, 132
  support group case study, 126, 132

Evenson, Mary E., 58, 59–77, 79
Experimental drugs, 155
Exposure-prone invasive procedures, 60, 69, 70, 71, 72, 74, 198
Express contracts, 179–180, 183, 184, 198
External forces, 2

F

Facility policies, 10
Facility procedures, 7
Facts, 122
Fadiman, Anne, *Spirit Catches You and You Fall Down, The,* 194
False entries, 90, 92, 94
False representation, 83
Family collaboration, 121, 138
Family Educational Rights and Privacy Act (FERPA), 13, 177
    background of, 22–23, 30
    cheating case study, 15–32
    confidentiality, 46
    HIV case study, 62, 63, 80
Family imposes treatment on relative case study, 152–163, 158–159, 160–163
Family needs, 142
Family therapy, 127
FBI. *See* Federal Bureau of Investigation
FDA. *See* Food and Drug Administration
Federal Bureau of Investigation (FBI), 22
Federal funding, 38
    and ADA, 37
    and HIV, 62, 74
    to hospitals, 37
    to universities, 28, 37
Federal institutions, Section 501 of the Rehabilitation Act of 1973, 40
Federally guaranteed student loans, 37, 38
Feminist Perspectives in Medical Ethics (Holmes and Purdy), 54
FERPA. *See* Family Educational Rights and Privacy Act
Fidelity to client, 94, 110
Fieldsteel, Nina, 84, 124, 125–130, 132
Fieldwork coordinators, 46
    and HIV challenges, 61–62
    memorandum of agreement, 61–62
    obligations of, 47
    rights and duties of, 55
Fieldwork placement, 39, 42
    emotional problems on fieldwork placement case study, 34–35, 46–49, 53–57
    fieldwork site requirements, 42–44, 49
    HIV case study, 70
    physical agent modalities, 105
    physical disability on fieldwork placement case study, 35, 49–52, 53–57
Fieldwork site requirements, 42, 198–199
Fieldwork supervisors, 51–52, 53, 55
Financial considerations, 121, 149
Fluidotherapy as physical therapeutic agent, 99
Food and Drug Administration (FDA) Code, 166
Frame of reference, physical agent modalities case study, 103, 199
Fraud, 90, 92, 93, 95
Functional independence, 121
Functional mobility, 119
Functional status, 133, 138, 143
Funding
    for health care, 5
    social planning, 7

G

"Gaming" the system, 146–148
    See also Lying versus gaming
Gaston v. Belhingrath Garden & Home, Inc., 48
Gates into practice, 58–81
Generalizations, 44, 50
Gilligan, C., 2
Gonzaga University, 17, 18, 19, 21
Gonzaga v. Doe, 17
Governmental intrusions on privacy rights, 21–22
Gracey, Colin B., 134, 164–173, 174
Graduate versus undergraduate levels, 25
"Greater good," 139
Group contract, 126–128
Group solidarity, 190
Groups
    confidentiality in, 84
    therapy in, 127
    See also Support group case study
Guardianship, 156–157, 159, 199
Gutheil, Thomas, 83, 85, 87–92, 95, 134, 152–159, 160, 189–193, 195
Gynecology, 60

H

Handicap, definition of, 38
Hansen, R., 29, 45
HBV. *See* Hepatitis B virus
HCFA. *See* Health Care Financing Administration
Health Care Financing Administration (HCFA), 114, 121
Health insurance. *See* Insurance
Health Insurance Portability and Accountability Act (HIPAA), 127, 167

Healthcare delivery
  bioethics in, 3–4
  HIV-infected healthcare workers, 70, 71, 74
  responsibilities of, 13
  studies on HIV and AIDS transmission, 67–68
Healthcare insurance, 3
Healthcare professions, 1, 4
Healthcare rationing. *See* Rationing of medical care; Rationing of treatment case studies
Healthcare resources, 14
Heat transfer, 100
Hepatitis B virus (HBV), 60, 66, 67, 74, 76
Hinojosa, Jim, 83, 97, 98–108
HIPAA. *See* Health Insurance Portability and Accountability Act
Hippocratic writings, 4
HIV. *See* Human immunodeficiency virus
HIV Prevention Strategic Plan through 2005, 64, 76
HIV/AIDS Bureau of the Health Resources and Services Administration, 62, 78
Holmes and Purdy, *Feminist Perspectives in Medical Ethics*, 54
Home health services, 121, 153, 161, 192
Homelessness, 159
Honesty, 30
Honor code, 30
Hospital policies, 10
Hot packs as physical therapeutic agent, 99
HRO. *See* Human Research Office
Human anatomy courses, 106
Human immunodeficiency virus (HIV), 127, 158, 199
  antibody test, 66, 74, 199
  case study, 13, 58–81
  confidentiality, 60, 62–63, 64, 65, 73
  emotional stability, 63–64
  ethical dilemma, 60
  evolving epidemic, 59–61
  fieldwork coordinator role, 61–62
  former client contact, 75
  incidence and prevalence statistics, 59–60, 67–68
  local guidelines, 69
  prevention interventions, 76–77
  professional guidelines, 68–69
  Recommendations for Post Exposure Prophylaxis (PEP), 68–69
  retrospective studies, 67–68
  risk of infection, 160
  safe-sex practices, 65
  testing for, 3, 13, 64–66, 74
    treatment services, 60, 65
    Universal Precautions, 66–67, 68, 69, 79
    university and federal guidelines, 69–75
    See also Acquired immunodeficiency syndrome (AIDS)
Human participant, 164–166, 169, 170, 173, 175, 199
Human Research Office (HRO), 166–167
Human rights of the individual, 2
Human subject, 164, 165, 168, 199

I

Immunizations of students, 61–62
Impairment, 36, 40–41, 199
Implied contracts (implied-in-fact), 179, 180, 184, 199
Improving the Quality of Nursing Home Care, Institutes of Medicine (IOM), 114
In-house versus out-of-house, 138
In loco parentis, 20, 21
Incompetence, 156–157
Independence, functional, 121
Independence versus gaining help from others, 54, 142
Independent living, 36
Indigent state hospital populations, 156–157
Individual differences, 125
Individual versus group treatment, 150–151
Individualized assessment, 50, 133
Individualized plans, 118
Infection control procedures, 67, 68–69, 72, 76
Infectious disease training programs, 70, 76
Information in informed consent, 154
Informative model of care, 160
Informed consent, 9, 61, 73, 110, 199
  bills of rights, 157
  bipolar disorder and ARC case study, 152–163, 157–158, 159–160
  competence, 153, 154–155, 161–162
  components of, 118–119
  definition, 154
  doctrine of consent to treatment, 154
  emergency exception, 155, 199
  family imposes treatment case study, 152–163, 158–159, 160–163
  guardianship, 156–157, 159
  See also Right to refuse treatment
Informed consent in research case study, 134, 164–175
  approval for research, 170
  Common Rule, 166, 167, 169, 170, 171

Informed consent in research case study, *(Continued)*
  confidentiality, 168, 169, 171, 172
  educational moments, 172
  guidelines for occupational therapy
    practitioner, 169–171
  Human Research Office (HRO),
    166–167
  human subject, 165
  institutional resources, 166–167
  medical data access, 168–169
  online courses, 170
  perception gap, 171
  principal investigator (PI), 168, 172, 174
  privacy, 168, 169
  Privacy Rule, 167
  reasons for diligence, 173
  regulations on human research, 167
  slippery slope and possible
    consequences, 172
  stakeholders, 167–168
Informed decisions, 9
Inner-city areas, 136, 148
Institutes of Medicine (IOM), *Improving
    the Quality of Nursing Home Care,*
    114
Institutional Compliance Division, 166
Institutional policies and procedures,
    166–167, 192
Institutional resources in research,
    166–167
Institutional Review Board (IRB), 166,
    168, 169, 170, 172, 173
"Institutional Review Board Management
    and Function" (Amdur and
    Bankert), 167
Insurance
  billable treatments, 92
  case studies, 85–87, 90, 91, 92–96, 151
  company policies, 7
  compensation by third-party payors, 88
  contracts with, 149
  and FERPA, 19
  "gaming" the system, 146–148
  medical, 3, 5
  uninsured and underinsured, 62–63
  uninsured versus insured people, 9, 44
  See also Third-party payors
Interdisciplinary assessment, 119
Internal moral code, 2
Internal Revenue Service (IRS), 22
Interpersonal processes, 103
Interpreters, 43
Interpretive model of care, 160
Invasion of privacy, 17
Invasive procedures, 60, 69, 70, 71, 72, 74
Involuntary treatment and/or

  hospitalization, 155
IRB. *See* Institutional Review Board
IRS. *See* Internal Revenue Service

J
Jaffee v. Redmond, 127
Job descriptions, 10
Job functions, essential, 51
Job retraining, 74
Job security in whistleblowing, 194
Joint Commission for the Accreditation of
    Health Care Organizations, 76
Justice, 9
  comparative, 7
  distributive, 7–8
  noncomparative, 7
Justice orientation, 2

K
Kohlberg, L., 2
Kornblau, Barbara L., 13, 34, 36–53, 56
Kyler-Hutchison, Penny
  analyzing ethical dilemmas, 45
  cheating case study, 15, 28–33
  client record case studies, 85, 92–96
  contracts case study, 176, 185–188
  human immunodeficiency virus (HIV)
    case study, 58, 78–80
  informed consent case studies, 152–163
  informed consent in research case
    study, 164, 173–175
  physical modalities case study, 97,
    108–111
  restraints in the nursing home case
    study, 112, 120–122
  students with disabilities case studies,
    34, 53–57
  support group case study, 124, 130–132
  whistleblower case study, 189, 193–195

L
Law, 44
  agency, 181, 184
  case, 156, 177
  civil, 177
  contract, 178–180, 182, 184
  definition, 4
  English common, 179
  and ethics, 44–45
Least restrictive and best environment,
    122
Legal capacity, 179, 180, 199
Legal consideration, 179
Legal dilemmas, 4, 199
Legal principles, 9–10
  reasonably prudent person theory, 10
Legality

physical agent modalities case study, 107
of subject matter in contracts, 179
Liability, 87, 111
  and client record, 87
  vicarious, 91, 92
Libel, 191
  definition, 25, 199
Licensing, 6, 44, 52, 137
  relicensure, 76
  standards for, 10
  state laws, 44, 83, 107, 111
Liebling, Linette, 77
Lifelong learning, 105
Light as therapeutic agent, 99
Litigation, 159
Local governments and ADA, 36, 37
Long-term facilities. *See* Restraints in the nursing home case study
Lying versus gaming, 147
  See also "Gaming" the system

M

Major life activities, 36, 41, 199
Maleficence, 6
Malpractice, 89, 90, 91
  defense against, 88, 111
Malpractice standards, 44
Managed care practices, 143, 149–150
Managers, 133–134
  contracts case study, 134, 176–188
  informed consent case studies, 134, 152–163
  informed consent in research case study, 134, 164–175
  rationing of treatment case studies, 133, 135–151
  whistleblower case study, 134, 189–195
  See also Supervisors
Mandated reporter in whistleblowing, 191, 199
Masculine culture, 54
Massachusetts Institute of Technology (M.I.T.) suicide case, 18–19, 21
Massachusetts State court system, 18
Measurement problems, 140, 141
Media attention, 75, 80
Mediation in whistleblowing, 193, 199
Medicaid, 5, 38, 113
  Centers for Medicare and Medicaid Services (CMS), 114, 121
Medical care, rationing of, 3
Medical data access, 168–169
Medical insurance. *See* Insurance, medical
Medical paternalism, 154, 160, 162
Medical practice, bioethics in, 3–4
Medicare, 5, 38, 52, 113

Centers for Medicare and Medicaid Services (CMS), 114, 121
Memorandum of agreement, 61–62
Mental health practice, 159
Mental illness, 153
  chronic mental disorders, 159
  and commitment/treatment schism, 155–156
  psychosis, 156
  See also Bipolar disorder and ARC case study
Mental impairments, 40–41
Minimum Data Set (MDS), 114–115, 199
Minorities, 156
Mobility
  functional, 119
  restriction of, 118
  See also Restraints in the nursing home case study
Modalities. *See* Physical agent modalities
Moral development, 2, 30
Moral dilemmas. *See* Ethical dilemmas
Morality, 3, 199
Morisky v. Broward County, 48
Multiple Project Assurances, Office of Human Research Protections (OHRP), 166
Mutual assent, 179, 180
Myths about restraint use, 117, 119

N

National Bioethics Advisory Commission, 166
National Board for Certification in Occupational Therapy (NBCOT), 32, 109, 111
National Coalition for Nursing Home Reform, 113–114
National origin (civil rights protection), 36
NBCOT. *See* National Board for Certification in Occupational Therapy
Need, principle of, 8
Negligence, 17
Nixon, Richard, 21
Noncomparative justice, principle of, 7
Nondiscrimination principles, 41–42, 62, 199–200
Nonmaleficence, principle of, 6, 83, 110, 133, 134, 187, 200
Non-state government employers with 15 or more employees and ADA, 37
Note signing case study, 86–87, 95–96
Note-takers, 43

Nursing Home Reform Act (NHRA), 113, 114, 115, 118
Nursing homes. *See* Restraints in the nursing home case study

O

Objective evidence, 50
Obligation to potential clients, 143–144
OBRA. *See* Omnibus Budget Reconciliation Act
Occupational Safety and Health Administration (OSHA), 76
Office of Civil Rights, 167
Office of Human Research Protections (OHRP), 172, 173
  Multiple Project Assurances, 166, 167
  online tutorials, 173
Office for Protection from Research Risks (OPRR), 168
Omnibus Budget Reconciliation Act (OBRA), 52, 84, 112–123, 200
Online courses, informed consent in research case study, 170, 173
Open-captioned videotapes, 43
OPRR. *See* Office for Protection from Research Risks
Oregon medical plan, 138, 140
OSHA. *See* Occupational Safety and Health Administration
Outside contracts, 44

P

Palliative care, 72
Paper trail, 192
Paperwork. *See* Client record; Documentation
Paraffin baths as physical therapeutic agent, 99
Parents
  dependent children status, 25
  surrogate, 20
Paternalism, medical, 154, 160, 162
Patients. *See* Clients
Patriarchal culture, 54
PEP. *See* Recommendations for Post Exposure Prophylaxis
Personal ethics, 132
Physical agent modalities case study, 83–84, 97–111, 200
  active versus passive processes, 102, 103
  competency, 105–107
  definitions, 99–100
  domain of concern of a profession, 101–103
  educational background, 103–105, 106
  frame of reference, 103

legality, 107
scope of practice, 100–103
thermal modalities, 99–100, 100t, 101t
tools, 98–99, 102, 103
  See also Tools of a profession
Physical disability on fieldwork placement case study, 35, 49–52, 53–57
Physical impairments, 40–41
Physical restraint, 200
  See also Restraints in the nursing home case study
Physician advocates, 138
Physicians' Desk Reference, 155
Physics courses, 106
PI. *See* Principal investigator
Plagiarism, 24, 26
Policy modifications, 42–43
Pollard v. Lyon, 26
Poole, Sally, 83
Postprofessional education, 104
Postsecondary institutions
  Section 504 of the Rehabilitation Act of 1973, 38, 39
  See also Universities
Potential clients, 143–144
Pregnant women, 64
Prejudice, 14, 49
Premarital sex, 79
Prima facie duty, 187
Principal investigator (PI), 168, 172, 174
Prioritizing services, 139–142
  sick/sicker clients for treatment, 145
  and third-party payors, 143
Prisoners, 156
Privacy rights, 9, 177, 200
  governmental intrusions on, 21–22
  informed consent in research case study, 168, 169
  invasion of, 17
  of students, 18, 19, 20, 21, 22, 23, 27, 28
  and technologic advances, 22
Privacy Rule, 167, 200
Private practice setting, 185
Pro bono work, 186
Professional commitment, 30
Professional ethics, 132
Professional organizations, 80
Professional responsibilities, 13
Professional standards, 7, 195
  and HIV, 60
Protection of society, 156
Protections in whistleblowing, 191–192, 200
Proxy decision making, 119
Public accommodations, 36, 37, 40, 46, 49, 200

Public clinics, 5
Public health guidelines on HIV, 60
Purposeful activities, 103

Q

Quality-of-care issues, 114, 121
"Quality of Well Being Scale" (Oregon), 140
Quasi-contracts (implied-in-law), 180, 184, 200

R

Race (civil rights protection), 36
Rationing of medical care, 3
Rationing of treatment case studies, 133, 135–151
  seven-day workweek, 136–137, 149–151
  too many cases to handle, 136, 145–148
    dilemma or not?, 147–148
    "gaming" the system, 146–148
  triage in an elder care facility, 135–136, 138–145, 148–149
    family needs, 142
    helping therapists make choices, 144
    obligation to potential clients, 143–144
    prioritizing care and third-party payors, 143
    prioritizing services, 139–142
    prioritizing sick/sicker clients for treatment, 145
    relative benefits, 139
    unsafe work environments, 148–149
Readily achievable changes for public accommodations, 40, 43, 200
Reasonable and accepted practice, 83, 134
  See also Customary practice
Reasonable accommodations, 47, 48, 49, 50–51
Reasonable payment in contracts, 183, 184, 200
Reasonably prudent person theory, 10, 162
Recommendations for Post Exposure Prophylaxis (PEP), 68–69
Records
  educational, 46, 63
  health, 63
  See also Client record; Documentation
Regulations governing nursing home care, 113–116
Regulations on human research, 167
Rehabilitation Act of 1973. *See* Section 504 of the Rehabilitation Act of 1973
Reimbursement case study, 85–86, 90, 92–95

Relative benefits, 139, 200
Relatives of clients, 138
Religion (civil rights protection), 36
Research
  bioethics in, 3–4
  and conflict of interests, 134
  funding for, 5, 37
  and informed consent, 134
Resident Assessment Instrument (RAI)/Minimum Data Set (MDS), 114–115, 200
Resident Assessment Protocols (RAPs), 115, 116t
Restraints in the nursing home case study, 84, 112–123
  alternatives to restraint, 116, 119, 120t, 122
  clinical decision making, 118–119
  patterns of restraint use, 117–118
    deleterious effects of physical restraint, 118, 118t
    rationale for restraint use, 117
    restraint-reduction initiatives, 117
  quality-of-care issues, 114, 121
  regulations governing nursing home care, 113–116
    historical perspective, 113–114
    Omnibus Budget Reconciliation Act (1987), 114
    physical restraint regulations, 115–116
    Resident Assessment Instrument (RAI)/Minimum Data Set (MDS), 114–115
    Resident Assessment Protocols (RAPs), 115, 116t
Retaliations in whistleblowing, 190, 191, 192, 195, 200
Right to refuse treatment, 57, 110, 134, 152, 155–157
Rights of oppressed, disenfranchised, or powerless populations, 156
Risk-benefit analysis, 88–89
Risk factors use of restraints, 117
Risk management approach, 83, 87
Role models, 52
Rotary International four-way test, 45

S

Sabol, Laurie, 77
Safe-sex practices, 69
Safety of clients, 49–52, 55, 57, 73
Safety requirements, Americans with Disabilities Act (ADA), 44
Sanctions, 44
"Sandwich generation," 161

"Scatter-gun approach." *See* "Shotgun approach"
Schwartzberg, Milton, 13, 15–28, 30, 134, 176–185
Schwartzberg, Sharan, 137–151
Scope of practice, physical agent modalities case study, 100–103
Section 501 of the Rehabilitation Act of 1973, federal institutions, 40
Section 504 of the Rehabilitation Act of 1973, 13, 36, 37–39, 40, 45, 46, 52, 74
    See also Americans with Disabilities Act
Self-care, 139
Self-determination, 8–9, 73, 84, 134
Senior centers, 161
Seroconversion, 66, 67
Seven-day workweek, 136–137, 149–151
    See also Rationing of treatment case studies
Sex (civil rights protection), 36
Sexual abuse, 127
Sexually transmitted disease clinics, 64
Sharp instruments, 68, 72
Shin v. Massachusetts Institute of Technology (M.I.T.), 18–19, 21
"Shotgun approach," 139–140, 142, 200–201
Sick/sicker clients treatments, 145
Signatures and record-keeping, 91–92
Skilled nursing facilities (SNFs), 113, 114
Slander, 26, 201
SNFs. *See* Skilled nursing facilities
Social contract ethics, 132
Social justice, 94
Social movements, 156
Social planning, 7
Social responsibility, 186
Social services, 121, 161
Social supports, 121
Society, competing needs of, 7, 133
Soft tissue, 99
Sound as therapeutic agent, 99
Southeastern Community College v. Davis, 38, 49
Specific competence, 162, 201
Spence v. Johnson, 25
Spirit Catches You and You Fall Down, The (Fadiman), 194
Splinting, 103
Standard measurements, 141
Standards for an Accredited Educational Program, Accreditation Council for Occupational Therapy (ACOTE), 104

Standards for Continuing Competence, American Occupational Therapy Association (AOTA), 104
Standards of Practice. *See* American Occupational Therapy Association (AOTA) Standards of Practice
"Standards for Privacy of Individually Identifiable Health Information" (Privacy Rule), 167
State governments and ADA, 36, 37
State hospital associations, 69
State licensure laws, 44, 107, 111
State public health departments, 69, 76
Stereotypes, 44, 49, 50
Student directory information, 22, 25
Students, 13–14
    cheating case study, 13, 15–32
    confidentiality of records, 22–23
    dependent children status, 25
    with disabilities, 13, 34–57
    emotional problems on fieldwork placement case study, 34–35, 46–49, 53–57
    federally guaranteed student loans, 37, 38
    HIV-infected healthcare workers, 70, 71, 74
    human immunodeficiency virus (HIV) case study, 13, 58–81
    physical disability on fieldwork placement case study, 35, 49–52, 53–57
    physical examinations and immunizations, 61–62
    privacy rights, 18, 19, 20, 21, 22, 23, 27, 28
    rights and duties of, 54–55
    suicide and privacy case, 18, 18–19, 21
Suicide and privacy case, 18, 18–19, 21
Supervisors
    credentialing trainees, 92
    signing off on treatment by assistants, 86–87
    ultrasound intervention case study, 97–111
    See also Clinicians; Managers
Support group case study, 84, 124–132
    agreement of confidentiality, 125, 131, 132
    boundary issues, 125, 128, 129, 130, 131
    definitions, 125–126
    dual relationships, 128
    ethical dilemmas, 125, 128–129
    ethics, 126, 132
    group contract, 126–128
    structure of the group, 126–128
Support networks, 80

Support strategies for whistleblowers, 192–193
Support and therapy groups
confidentiality in, 84
See also Support group case study
Surrogate parenthood, 3, 20

T
Tarasoff decision, 127
Technologic advances, 98, 100, 101
and privacy rights, 22
in treatment, 4, 105
Telecommunications, 36
devices for the deaf, 43
Temperature as therapeutic agent, 99
Theoretical background. *See* Ethical
dilemmas; Ethical principles; Legal
dilemmas; Legal principles
Therapy groups, confidentiality in, 84
Thermal modalities, 99, 99–100, 100t,
101t, 201
Third-party payors, 143, 144, 146, 150,
201
See also Insurance
Threshold effect, 139
Too many cases to handle, 136, 145–148
See also Rationing of treatment case
studies
Tools of a profession, 98–99, 102, 103,
150, 201
See also Physical agent modalities case
study
*Toyota Motor Mfg., Kentucky, Inc. v.
Williams*, 41
Transfer techniques, 119
Transportation, 36
Triage in an elder care facility, 135–136,
138–145, 148–149
See also Rationing of treatment case
studies
TRI-CARE/CHAMPUS, 38
Trudeau, Scott, 84, 112, 113–120
True contracts, 179
Trust, 30, 56
in groups, 127, 130
in human research system, 173
Tufts University, 77

U
Ultrasound intervention case study,
97–111
Ultrasound as physical therapeutic agent,
99
Unconscious bias, 14
United States Department of Education,
27–28, 38
United States Department of Health and

Human Services, 166, 167
United States Department of Justice, 38,
45, 48, 52
United States Public Health Service, 69
United States Supreme Court
Gonzaga v. Doe, 17, 19
Jaffee v. Redmond, 127
judges in, 4
Universal Precautions, 14, 66, 67, 68, 158,
159, 201
Universal Precautions for Prevention and
Transmission of HIV, HBV, and
Other Bloodborne Pathogens in
Health Care Settings (CDC),
66–67
Universities
federal funding to, 28
graduate versus undergraduate levels,
25
internal investigations, 24, 26–27
legal counsel, 23–24, 28
policies and procedures, 16, 23, 24, 25,
30
responsibilities of, 13
See also Postsecondary institutions
University counseling centers, and HIV
counseling, 64
Unsafe work environments, 148–149
Utilitarianism, 186–187, 201
Utility, principle of, 6–7, 133, 134, 201
Utilization review, 88, 89, 92

V
Values, 3, 29, 61, 122
Veracity or truth telling, 30, 110, 111
Verbal agreements, 179
Veterans Administration, 37, 39–40
Vicarious liability, 91, 92, 201
Videotext displays, 43
Volume-control telephones, 43
Voluntariness, 154–155
Voluntary disclosure, 70, 71

W
Wards of the state, 156–157
Washing hands and infection control
precautions, 68
Washington State, 17
Water as therapeutic agent, 99
Watergate hearings, 21
Wendell, Susan, 54
Whirlpool baths as physical therapeutic
agent, 99
Whistleblowers, 90, 92, 94, 189–195, 201
alternatives to, 192
case study, 189–190
disinterested parties, 191

Whistleblowers *(Continued)*
  documentation, 192–193
  institutional policies and procedures,
    192
  mandated reporter, 191
  mediation, 193
  protections, 191–192
  retaliations, 190, 191, 192, 195
  role of, 190–191
  support strategies, 192–193

  witnesses and consultants, 193
Witnesses and consultants in
  whistleblowing, 193
Work environments, unsafe, 148–149
Work opportunities, 159
Written consent, 61, 63, 70, 73
Written contract, 176–177, 178, 184
  See also Contracts
Written guidelines, 84
Wrongful death suit, 18